Making it Happen

Every day somebody helps me in some way. From a stranger helping me cross a busy road, to a close friend racing with me in a sports event, from the associates who assist me with my business interests, to the many, many people who are there for me day to day. I worry that I have not said thank you to every single person who has helped me along the way.

It is to these people that I dedicate this book.
You know who you are and I thank you!

Making it Happen

MARK POLLOCK

with ROSS WHITAKER

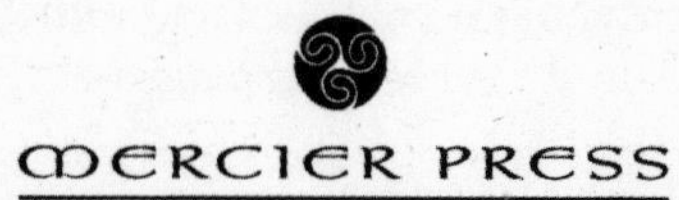

MERCIER PRESS
Douglas Village, Cork, Ireland
www.mercierpress.ie

Trade enquiries to Columba Mercier Distribution,
55a Spruce Avenue, Stillorgan Industrial Park, Blackrock, Dublin

ISBN 1 85635 487 3

10 9 8 7 6 5 4 3 2 1

Front cover photograph of Mark Pollock (right) and John O'Regan (left) at the finishing line of the North Pole 2004 marathon reproduced by kind permission of www.northpolemarathon.com. © *Mike King.*

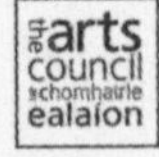

Mercier Press receives financial assistance from the Arts Council/An Chomhairle Ealaíon

Printed and Bound by J. H. Haynes & Co. Ltd, Sparkford

CONTENTS

ACKNOWLEDGEMENTS

Mark and Ross would each like to thank their family and friends who have been so incredibly supportive over the years. There are truly too many to mention in a book, let alone a page.

We would also specifically like to thank all of the contributors to this book and everyone else who helped us to 'make it happen'.

FOREWORD

COURAGE IN THE FACE OF adversity is something we should all aspire to, as well as admire.

For Mark Pollock, everything in life was going wonderfully well. He was in his final year at Trinity College Dublin where he was studying Business Studies and Economics. He was rowing for Trinity, had a job offer from an investment bank and had recently celebrated his twenty-second birthday.

And then, quite suddenly, he had to face the trauma and the terror of losing his sight. That was in 1998.

It was in February 1999 that I got to know Mark. He came to work with us at IAWS Group for a year. In so many respects he was an inspiration to everyone with whom he came in contact. His ability, his willingness to be a team player and his 'can do' attitude were his hallmarks.

In *Making It Happen* Mark declares: 'In the last seven years I have been greatly challenged by things that I would never have expected to be challenged by.' This book stands as an inspiration to us all. In his own words: 'this book is about moving from the "making excuses" category to the "making it happen" category.'

Here you will find what they don't teach you in university: the education that is garnered from what is euphemistically called 'the university of life'. Mark's qualifications for writing this book are his experiences. For this very reason, his book, which deals with acceptance, changing one's life to cope with circumstances, altering course, setting and achieving goals and team playing, is as inspiring as it is interesting.

Finally, I commend and congratulate those who stood loyally by Mark during those difficult times and who gave him the encouragement, the nurturing and the love which have sustained him.

Philip Lynch
Managing Director, IAWS
2004

1

LEARNING TO TAKE CONTROL

THIS BOOK IS FOR everyone who wants to get more from their life: from those who have yet to take the first step towards the life they want, to those who are on the cusp of achieving everything they have ever dreamed of.

This book combines my story and the story of others. In writing it I have spoken to people about what they have done to make the most of their lives. I have spoken with people who have achieved many successes and people who have achieved few. They have told me about overcoming obstacles, taking on challenges, showing determination and changing their lives for the better. This book is about all of those people. It is about people who have tried for years to succeed and it is about people who are just embarking on their first journey. It is about my friends and acquaintances, about people I have met on my travels and at conferences and business meetings. It is about me. Perhaps it is about you.

As you will find out in this book, I have faced some major difficulties in my life and I have had to use all of my physical, mental and emotional resources to keep my life on track. I lost my sight a number of years ago and since then I have thought hard about how people overcome adversity and make the most of their lives. I became blind in 1998. At the time,

I was on the crest of a wave; everything was going my way. I was about to finish a Business Studies and Economics degree in Trinity College Dublin. My studies were going well and I was confident of making it through my final exams. To be honest, I hadn't always done well in university. In fact, I had struggled in the first two years but by my final year I felt I was on top of things and, as far as I was concerned, that was an achievement in itself.

Other aspects of my life were also going well. I was rowing for my university and wanted to further progress my international sporting career. I had rowed for Ireland as a junior and had just missed out on going to the World Championships in 1997 but I hoped to be able to row for Ireland at future World Championships. In addition, I had a job offer from an investment bank in London and my plan was to start work after graduation. Everything was really going my way. The sky was the limit and I was in flight.

Then everything changed. In the space of two short weeks I changed from someone who knew exactly who I was and where I was going into someone who didn't know if I had any future at all. The academic, sporting and work-related factors upon which I had based my identity all vanished when I lost my eyesight. My identity vanished with them. My future had seemed so bright but now I was in darkness. Complete darkness.

It wasn't the first time that I had had problems with my eyes. I lost the sight in my right eye following a detached retina at the age of five and went on to have a number of operations on my 'good' left eye. So I was no stranger to the succession of hospital beds and doctors' waiting-rooms that went along with that. Despite this, at no stage in my life did I ever really face the possibility that I might some day become blind.

It was never on the agenda. I didn't even contemplate it. I knew that if I got hit on the head I might develop another detached retina but the doctors had always been able to fix them in the past and I had no reason to believe that they wouldn't continue to do so in the future.

But on 10 April 1998, two weeks after first noticing blurred vision in my left eye during a rowing training session, I started a journey that was to be the beginning of my new life.

The journey began in April but it wasn't until mid July that year, after two failed operations, that I was finally told that I would not see again. Between April and July I was in limbo; unable to face blindness head on, but at the same time having no choice but to put my normal life on hold. As I slowly began to realise that I was going to remain blind, I also started to realise that my previous identity no longer existed. The horror of being relegated to the 'disabled' bin was too awful for words; I felt my life was over. Everything that had defined me was gone forever and I didn't know myself any longer.

Since that day I have been greatly challenged by things that I would never have expected to be challenged by. The first challenge was getting out of bed. Next was finding my way around the house, dressing myself and learning to read my watch. Later, I moved on to living on my own, getting a job and doing a master's degree, and more recently I have relaunched my sporting career and started my own business. When I was dealing with blindness as a possibility, I didn't think I would be able to do any of these things.

It almost sounds easy, even to me, when I recount the story of the last few years, but the reality is that it wasn't easy. I think I have been through every emotion known to man. It has been a difficult journey and one that has taken me to a place I never expected. My life now is so far detached from what I thought it would be that I struggle to even describe my feelings during the period immediately following my going blind.

Seven years have passed since that frightening moment when I lost my sight and I am happy to be able to say that I now view my blindness as an inconvenience rather than a life stopping disability. So much of what I thought was impossible back then wasn't impossible at all. Obstacles that seemed insurmountable were overcome with time and effort and, with each obstacle that I have overcome, life has become better.

But this book is not just about me. This book is about taking control of our life journeys and making the most of life.

As I became more firmly in control of my life, I began to realise how many people around me seemed to allow themselves to be controlled by someone or something other than themselves. A lot of people seemed to be dissatisfied with the events in their lives and yet were doing nothing to improve matters. Every now and then I would meet someone who was in control of his or her life and I began to wonder what the difference was. I had gone from one category to the other in quite a short space of time so it really fascinated me. This book is about just that, moving from the 'making excuses' category to the 'making it happen' category.

For this book, I decided to go out and find people who could shed light on the subject. I wanted to find real stories and concrete examples that would help me and others to better understand what it takes to make good things happen in life. Having spoken to many such people I have found common themes that link them and I have tried, where possible, to draw conclusions and link them in a way that you might find helpful. I should make it clear that I interviewed each person as an individual as part of my research and that all of the conclusions I reached are my own. I learned a lot from them and I hope you will too.

Their stories show how important it is to take responsibility for your life. I know we have all heard that before but the truth of it has really struck me in talking to successful people. It is a theme that is repeated often in the conversations I have had with them and it is an important theme of this book. The people I have met 'own' their lives in a way that many people don't. They make their decisions based on what they think is best, rather than allowing other parties to dictate to them. Regardless of their circumstances, they have continued to take responsibility for themselves and their happiness. By making that their priority, they have invariably achieved a life they enjoy.

I am not a sociologist or a psychologist and I would never claim to be. My qualifications for writing this book are my experiences, my journey. Also, I have spent the last few years going to companies and giving motivational lectures. In this time I have heard so many stories that I have begun to understand the difference between successful and unsuccessful people. I feel it is worth documenting this information in the hope that it might be useful to others.

Because my qualifications for writing this book are my experiences, I will be framing the chapters around my own journey. People always advise writers to write what they know and I know nothing better than I know my life. The first and most important thing that I was forced to do was to accept my circumstances and that is the first thing, I think, that everyone must do. In my case, it was particularly hard, but in the end inevitable. One can't deny blindness forever! While becoming blind is never easy, it is a very cut-and-dried situation and in a way that's a blessing, not a curse. For many people living seemingly normal lives it is hard for them to accept that, in reality, they are not in control of their lives.

So acceptance is the first thing I will discuss. After that, I will look at how we can make the first steps towards changing our lives so that we are more in control. Chapter four will look at making things happen as opposed to making excuses. There are times in our journey where we must decide whether to persist with the thing that we have set out to do or change emphasis and concentrate on something new and I will look at that in chapter five. Chapter six is about setting and achieving goals and chapter seven is about forming a team around you to help you in life.

That is the path I have taken to move from a situation where my life was not my own, to one where I now feel that I am living the life I want to. I now feel that I *own* my life. It is important for people who are in a position to do so to take ownership of their lives. It took me six years to move from chaos to control and in this book I will explain the path I took. Others I have spoken to have gone through some similar experiences, but also some very different ones that I hope you will find helpful.

2

WHERE AM I? FINDING THE BIG RED DOT

I'M SURE YOU'VE HEARD it said that every journey begins with the first step. That sounds very nice but I'm not sure that I agree with it. I think every journey begins with some planning. I'm not necessarily suggesting that you plan everything and, indeed, in some of the best journeys the first step is made with no particular destination in mind. But every journey must start with the decision to make that journey and a decision as to which direction that first step will take. Of course to take this first step you must first know where you are.

Most of us have done it. We have opened a map and planned a journey from A to B. First we look at where we are, A, then we look at where we want to go, B, and finally we plan a course between them. Sometimes when we are in a strange country or a new city we have trouble even locating A. Maps in towns or in museums often have that big red dot that says 'You are Here' and this gives us the starting point from which we make our plan. It's relatively easy to get around in this way.

When we are planning our life journeys it is a little bit more difficult than that. There is no big red dot that says 'You are Here' and there is no map that will guarantee that we will make it from A to B. This chapter is about finding the 'big red dot' that tells you where you are. As soon as you have found it you will be ready to take that first step on your journey.

Ironically, one can undergo quite a journey just to find the 'big red dot'. There are many pressures – emotional, environmental, time, family, to name a few – that can make it difficult to figure out who you are and where you are. Once you do find and accept the reality or your current situation, then you are ready to take that all-important first step.

The Model

In 1969, Elizabeth Kubler-Ross wrote a book called *On Death and Dying* that was based on her research on the grief process. Her book helped to popularise the view that the process can be represented in steps or stages. While her research was concerned with the reaction of grieving people to the loss of loved ones, my experience is that it can equally be applied to many other situations. First though I will explain the stages that Kubler-Ross outlined in relation to grieving.

- The first stage is denial. In the model, people deny death because they are unable to admit to themselves that the patient has died, or will die, and that they will suffer loss as a result.
- The second stage is anger. Typically at this stage a person projects his or her pain onto others, becoming angry and blaming others for the situation.
- The next stage is called 'bargaining'. Bargaining represents a last effort at overcoming death by 'earning' a longer life. At this point people sometimes attempt to make a deal with God in which they will receive some kind of miracle in return for good behaviour.
- The fourth stage is depression or self-pity, which occurs

when the likelihood of death, or the death itself, has sunk in and the person is overcome with sadness.

- The final stage is acceptance. At this stage the grieving person comes to grips with the fact of the patient's death and makes preparations for it.

We must first arrive at a point where we accept our current reality before we are able to take the next step in our lives. When I think about my own life and discuss with others the highs and lows of their lives it becomes clear to me that this model can apply to small challenges or giant obstacles both in our work and outside of it. Often we experience some or all of the stages before we finally accept our situation and move on. Let's look at some of the stages in the model and see how they can relate to everyday life.

Denial

Denial is the first stage. We've heard it so many times, indeed people often throw it in with the bar banter. One man might say to his friend: 'I'm not going to ask that girl out, I'm not attracted to her at all.' And his friend will promptly reply: 'Obviously you do like her. You've been talking about her all night. You're just in denial.' This kind of chat would have you believe that denial is an everyday thing and I think it is but it is still quite dangerous. Denial can prevent us understanding the truth of a situation and acting on it. It is a way of not admitting to ourselves that we have a problem so that we avoid the problem entirely. But if we deny our problems then we end up running away from them instead of confronting them.

When I became blind I was in denial for four months. In a way that might seem strange because my reality was obvious – I simply could not see. I was in darkness yet I would not get a white stick or apply for a guide dog. I didn't want to be blind and I denied it because I didn't want it to be true. If you close your eyes right now you will understand that it is difficult to deny that you can't see even when the world around you is completely black. Despite living in this kind of darkness all day, every day, I still managed to deny it. If it is possible to deny something as obvious as complete darkness then it is possible to deny things that are much less obvious than that.

I know that I have experienced similar denial in other parts of my life. In my sporting endeavours, I have sometimes not faced up to the fact that I am not doing the level of training necessary to compete at the level that I want to be at. In my studies, I have at times not faced the fact that I was not doing the level of work required to get the results I desired. I have been in denial at work too and not faced the reality that I was not doing the job that I really wanted to do. Denial is part of my world and part of many people's worlds.

It is amazing how easy it is to be in denial and how often we do it. If there is a person out there who has never been in denial then I haven't met him or her. Denial is the outright rejection of one's reality. That sounds very drastic and the truth is that in day-to-day life denial isn't quite that drastic. Perhaps, for instance, you want a new job but you are waiting in your current job because you don't want to leave your company in the lurch. Perhaps the job you really want to do pays less and you are just saving a little bit more until you make the switch. Maybe you would love to learn to play the guitar or to get in shape, but you just can't find the time right now, even though you watch several hours of television a week. Maybe you would like to give more money to charity but you just don't feel like you have the extra money to give away even though your life is comfortable.

The truth of the matter is that when we do this we are rejecting the reality that we are not doing the things that we actually want to do. We are not doing the job we want to do, we are not spending our time in the way that we want to and we are not spending our money in the way that we want to. In short, we do not have the life that we want.

Denial is a way of dealing with the disappointment of your life not being the way that you want it to be.

It can be very comforting. Telling yourself that you will change to the job you want just as soon as you've saved enough money for a new car is comforting because the intention to change jobs is there. Telling yourself that you would have won the gold medal if you had prepared better is comforting because in your mind you were good enough to have won the gold medal. In both of these situations your confidence remains intact because you have denied the reality of the situation. The truth is that you are not in the job you want and you did not win the gold medal.

How many times have you not admitted that you avoided the truth of a given situation? How many times have you buried your head in the sand, unwilling to stare the facts straight in the face and deal with them? How many times have you made excuses? These are difficult questions to answer. Sometimes the answer can be upsetting. Don't be disheartened though, because once you have figured this out you are on the road to finding that job and winning those medals, if these are the things that you want to do. To illustrate this, let me tell you the story of a young man I met called Gavin.

Gavin wanted to be a doctor from the age of ten. His grandfather, with whom he was very close, was a doctor, as was his uncle, and his mother was a nurse, so there was a strong medical history in the family. In secondary school he did all of the science subjects – physics, chemistry and biology – but he didn't get the grades necessary to get into medicine. Despite the fact that he was only sixteen years old he decided not to repeat his final year in school in an effort to get into medicine. He went to university and studied maths. After a couple of years, he switched to maths and economics. He thought about medicine at that point but decided it would be too expensive and that he was too old to go back. He was nineteen at that stage. He plodded on through university and finished with a degree in maths and economics, despite the fact that he never really enjoyed the subjects.

Next, he did a master's degree in economics. He studied hard and got good grades. Not sure that he wanted to be an economist, he got a job teaching in Asia. It was great fun but he didn't want to do it for a career. He was now aged twenty-three and wondered what he might do next. At the end of the year in Asia, he got the medicine application forms for college but never filled them out. He decided once again that it was too late to go back. He decided that apart from medicine the only other thing that could motivate him was money. He had seen the lavish lifestyles of the rich ex-pats in Singapore and decided to go for that. He studied for a master's degree in financial mathematics in Edinburgh University and was offered a lucrative job with UBS in the city of London as a foreign exchange strategist. Later he became a trader and was recruited by the world's biggest bank, Citibank. He was successful there and from the outside his lifestyle looked fantastic, but he wasn't entirely happy. His boss was offered a promotion and as a vote of confidence, Gavin's boss offered Gavin his job. That was the day that Gavin quit.

His boss thought about offering him more money to stay but he knew that Gavin's decision was made. At the age of twenty-nine he had finally decided to go back and study medicine. For years Gavin had placed obstacles on the path between himself and medicine. He had told himself many times that he was too old and that it was too expensive. He knew that going back and doing medicine would be a hard road, so he had told himself that it wasn't that important to him and that other things could satisfy him. Fortunately he was smart enough to realise that he did really want to do medicine so he stopped denying his dissatisfaction with his situation and did something about it. In the end he overcame the denial and decided to do the thing he really wanted to do. He is so happy that he did.

Anger and Blame

Once people stop denying the reality of their situation, they begin to realise that their life isn't all they thought it was. Not surprisingly, a lot of people get angry. When we realise that our situation is not the way we would like it to be, our instinct can be defensive. Such defensive feelings can manifest themselves in angry reactions. Rather than taking time to evaluate the situation and decide what to do next we express anger externally or bottle it up inside.

During the early months while denying my blindness I was angry with the people who were trying to help me. I remember a guy from the social services came to help me with my rehabilitation. His name was Barry and his job was to teach me how to cook. The first thing we did was what is known in the rehabilitation services as 'hob management'. I was being taught how to boil a pot of water without burning myself. I remember being utterly appalled that I, a potential high-flyer (at least in my mind!), was going through the indignity of being taught how to boil a pot of water at the age of twenty-two.

Throughout the hob-management lesson I was fuming inside. I didn't say anything to Barry because I didn't want to undermine his job. However, I suspect that he knew I was angry because I was neither enthusiastic nor overly appreciative. Suffice to say we never went near the cooker again. I was angry with Barry for having to be there at all but throughout his visits I spent more time cursing other people and in particular the government departments who were making it difficult for me to access services by delaying, making me fill in forms and generally insisting that I go through 'the process'. Barry, my family, friends and the departments themselves put up with my outbursts. I moaned about other people and blamed them. I got a sore head from the stress. I cried in my room and hit the wall and pillow. I was very angry, but it passed. Of course, with hindsight, I know Barry was actually helping me, but at the time I could not get over the fact that I didn't want him to be there at all, never mind teach me how to boil a pot of water.

Anger is often inextricably linked to blame: blaming our colleagues, friends, family, society, governments or anyone else that might be in the firing line. When we are in this phase we ask: 'Why should this happen to me?' or 'How could you let this happen? Why can't you help?' Allowing ourselves to externalise these questions and put the blame on someone else helps us to cope with the issues without actually facing up to them.

It is unusual for us to be in a rage about the events of our lives. It is more usual for us to blame others for the reality of our lives. It is very easy to focus on other people when we are not achieving what we want. I have a friend who was a student in university around the same time as me. He was preparing for one of his final exams when he noticed that certain topics came up on the exam every year. In this particular paper students had to answer four questions out of ten and he figured there were four topics that recurred every year. While more conservative students took a broad approach to the course, he decided to become an expert in those four topics. On the day of the exam only two of his questions were on the paper and he barely scraped a pass. To this day he blames the lecturer. The person who came top of the class isn't blaming anyone.

Things in life don't always go our way and most of us understand that this is the way of the world. We win some and we lose some. If we take credit for the victories then we must take responsibility for the defeats. At least, we shouldn't blame other people for them. I learned after a while that there was no reason to be angry with Barry or anyone else. And there was no need to be angry with myself either. Reality is nobody's fault, it just exists and there's no sense in being angry about it. Sometimes our anger and fixation with blaming other people detract from the business of moving on. The sooner that we take responsibility for our ambitions and stop focusing on how other people might be interfering with our mission in life, the sooner we are in a position to move forward.

Are you blaming somebody right now for the fact that you are not achieving the things you want? Take responsibility yourself and realise that you are the only one who can change your situation.

Searching for Miracles

But how do we move forward? Well, firstly we look for a miracle. It is much easier to look for a miracle than to have to actually deal with a problem. Sometimes this is when people remember religion. People might ask: 'God, if I'm a good Christian, will you sort this out for me?' I am not a scholar of theology, but the small amount I have learned about religion suggests that this is not how God works. He doesn't give guarantees that you will get the job that you covet and he certainly won't find you a husband or wife or build a house for you.

I was not religious prior to going blind and I am still not. I did, however, have a period of pleading with God to help me. I remember after about three months of being blind I was lying in bed awake in the middle of the night with my eyes open and seeing nothing. For a brief moment I saw what I thought was the head of Jesus. I thought it could have been the type of sign that you hear people talking about. Was it a sign or a trick of the mind? In any case, when I woke up the next day, I still couldn't see. For a moment that night, perhaps, I thought that God might restore my sight and everything would be back to normal, but it wasn't. That night I was searching for a miracle.

Although people often turn to God in these moments, I don't think there necessarily needs to be a religious slant to this search for miracles. This phase can be characterised by something as simple as hoping for a bit of good luck. We have all, at times, relied on perceived luck or hoped for some coincidence that allows us achieve a result that does not necessarily tally with the effort we have put in. We often hope or pray for outcomes that in reality are completely outside our control. I knew a girl once who wanted to be a dancer. She said categorically that if she could be what she really wanted to be then she would be a dancer. Although she was doing absolutely nothing to further this aim she still hoped that it would happen. She was hoping, in effect, for a miracle. She is still not a dancer.

Contrast this with the story of the famous golfer from South Africa, Gary Player. It is over forty years since he came onto the world golf scene. It didn't take him long to make an impact. He was talented and fiercely competitive but more than anything he had an incredible drive to make himself better. He was one of the most diligent workers that the golf driving range had ever seen and he recognised the importance of fitness in golf long before Tiger Woods made it fashionable. Player's talent and diligence made him one of the greatest golfers to ever play the game. Funnily enough when he first started to become successful some observers thought he was just lucky. Player had the perfect answer. He said: 'The more I practise, the luckier I get.' It might sound like a cliché but we have to make our own luck in life. Miracles can happen, but I wouldn't recommend waiting around for one.

A friend of mine by the name of Conor is another good example of someone who is not prepared to wait for a miracle to happen and has decided to make his own luck. When Conor was growing up he was obsessed with sailing. It was the most important thing in his life and he never really thought about school. He went to university and studied science, but really this was just because his peers were doing it. His main focus was always sailing and when he started university he soon realised that he had no interest in studying. He scraped through university, at no point being inspired by what he was doing.

Conor wasn't just interested in sailing, he was good at it too. He was a member of the National Youth Development Team but towards the end of his time in college the team was disbanded and he didn't have the financial resources to pursue an Olympic campaign. Disheartened, he gave up competitive sailing. Studying a course that didn't interest him and no longer sailing, Conor worried that he might be condemned to a life of mediocrity so he started to think of other things he could do. In science he had been interested in the body and he thought about doing dentistry because he also liked working with his hands. He applied for dentistry but wasn't accepted.

Conor felt that this was a make or break time for him and he thought long and hard about what to do. He decided to apply for dentistry again a year later, but this time he didn't just apply to one school, he applied to them all. He was invited for an interview and this time he was accepted. He feared that he would struggle because he was surrounded by some of the most gifted students in the country so he worked hard and for the first three years finished solidly in the middle of his class. He was enjoying his studies and the more he got into it the more it became a replacement for sailing, a replacement for that competitive edge that he used to enjoy. He began to aim higher.

At the end of his third year in dentistry he made a thirteen-year plan. He looked at what he was doing from the outside and identified what he would have to do to achieve the things he wanted. He wanted to be an oral and maxillofacial surgeon, which is one of the most difficult things to achieve in dentistry. He decided that he would leave no stone unturned in his quest to achieve his goals but he could see that there were what he calls 'bottle-necks' along the way. These are points where he recognised there would be very few positions available and the demand would be high. When there were only three positions available as a house officer upon completing his degree, Conor prepared as if there was only one position. He tried to make failure impossible and he succeeded.

He did the same at the next 'bottle-neck' when he was applying for an accelerated medicine course. To make himself more attractive he submitted and had published articles in dental/medical journals and did courses normally only attended by qualified doctors. He was accepted everywhere he applied.

He wasn't prepared to rely on luck – he made his own luck.

I think Conor is quite unique in that he is so incredibly focused on achieving the things he has set his mind to. I was taken aback by the vigour with which he has pursued his goals and I found it particularly amazing because I remember a time when he wasn't quite so focused. In the meantime he hasn't fundamentally changed. His biology is still the same. His genetics haven't changed. The changes that have occurred have been in finding something that he really enjoyed doing and in making his own luck. These are things that any of us can do.

Are you waiting for a miracle? Maybe it's time to start making your own luck.

Self-pity

Often when we realise that a miracle won't save us we can become affected in an emotional way. You might never have been diagnosed with depression in your life but you have probably felt self-pity at some point. I think we have all felt sorry for ourselves now and again. I have certainly experienced prolonged feelings of loss and unhappiness related to the serious business of becoming blind. I have also felt sorry for myself in more mundane moments of my life. There have even been times when I have successfully achieved goals but then realised that they were not the right goals and felt sorry for myself as a result.

Helen Keller once said that 'Self-pity is our worst enemy and if we yield to it, we can never do anything wise in this world'. Self-pity is a drug that is addictive. It is a very easy rut to get stuck in and a very hard rut to get out of. The result of self-pity is that we become paralysed and unable to do anything else. Self-pity can grip people for many years and it is something that is very frightening and divisive. To people who are suffering from depression, I have nothing to say because I am not qualified to do so and this is not really the place to discuss it anyway. What I am talking about here is a level of self-pity that can be identified and rectified by an individual.

We all feel sorry for ourselves from time to time and it is something that really serves no productive purpose. In some cases it is just something we have to go through and the challenge is to recognise that it is happening and to drag ourselves out of it. Are you feeling sorry for yourself at the moment? Is it stopping you from doing something? I could feel sorry for myself right now because it is late at night and I want to finish off this chapter soon so I can get some sleep. Feeling sorry for myself won't get me to bed any quicker, so I'm better off accepting it and getting on with it. The thing that leads us out of self-pity is finding acceptance. When we have finally accepted our situation then we can do something about it.

Acceptance

In the Kubler-Ross model, the fifth and final stage is acceptance. When we reach acceptance we have reached a true understanding of the problem, difficulty or challenge facing us. Only by accepting the good, the bad and the ugly in our lives can we make any progress. In many ways acceptance can be more difficult than denial. Living in reality can be more difficult than living in the unreal comfort zone that we have built for ourselves. However, as soon as we accept reality, we can move forward and build a life far more satisfying than any comfort zone we could ever create. When we have reached acceptance we have reached the 'big red dot' that I described earlier. At this point we can say, 'I am here'. We can look at the map of our journey, find A and start planning our trip to B and beyond. We must all go through at least some of the stages outlined in this chapter before we can reach acceptance.

I recently read the story of Tony Adams on the internet and he is a great example of someone who went through a lot before reaching acceptance. He was one of England's most successful footballers ever. He was a real winner and became an Arsenal Football Club legend, captaining them to several trophies. His drinking also gained him legendary status. During the 1990–91 football season, with Arsenal heading towards their second league title in three years, Adams was jailed for a drink-driving offence. A few years later he publicly admitted he was an alcoholic and entered rehabilitation.

The Tony Adams who emerged was a different man. He continued to give his all for Arsenal but his reaction to victories and defeats had changed. He still wanted to win every game, but he now felt that it was in giving each game his all that he would achieve victory. If the team lost, he would accept it and move on to thinking of the next game. His teammates found it difficult to understand but Adams' experiences with addiction had given him a new balance. His self-esteem wasn't based on the highs of victory or the lows of defeat anymore, but on the fact that he was now in control of his life. He had decided before the game had ever begun that he was a winner. He had taken control of his life and reached the point of acceptance.

I certainly went through all of the stages before reaching acceptance. My family and friends were incredibly helpful but soon they all started to get on with their own lives. This is, of course, understandable and, anyway, I slowly started to realise that no matter how much my mum, my dad or my sister Emma attempted to make my life as easy as possible, they couldn't live my life for me, nor did I want them to. And at the same time I couldn't live my life through my friends who were starting jobs in London, travelling around the world or representing their country in sport. I wanted to be doing all of these things but I wasn't doing any of them.

Instead, my life was becoming defined by drinking too much, lying in bed until lunchtime or beyond, listening to talk radio and generally enduring life rather than living it. Feelings of anger, loneliness and fear soon gave way to intense boredom. It rapidly became clear that no longer could I deny the blindness, no longer was there any point in being angry, and no longer was there any value in bargaining to get better or wallowing in self-pity. I decided to draw a line under the issue and accept that I was blind.

As soon as I faced the seemingly horrible truth – the facts of my new life – it didn't seem so bad. I immediately moved on. I started using a white stick. A small point you might think but actually holding a white stick and admitting to yourself that you are 'one of those people' is very difficult. The problem wasn't even just admitting it to myself. I also felt an overwhelming paranoia that everyone was looking at me. In contrast, the reality was that people stopped calling me an idiot when I bumped into them and I didn't feel so weird holding onto my male friend's arms when going to the bathroom in bars!

Soon after I got my white stick, I battled to get on a computer course so that I could learn how to use the equipment that I have used to write this book. You see, as soon as I had accepted my blindness I was energised to make the most of my life. I spoke to the Royal National Institute for the Blind in Belfast but they didn't have a computer course for six months. My complete lack of patience, coupled with a passionate desire to get started on my new life helped me to look at other options.

I found a training school with a suitable course and contacted my local government agency which had the power to put me on the course if there were places. However, after a series of follow-up calls from me to the department with no response I took matters into my own hands. Having established that a place was available immediately, I contacted the area supervisor of the government department that I had been dealing with and explained the urgency of my situation and my enthusiasm for getting approval to begin the course. That evening I met a representative from the Royal National Institute for the Blind in a hotel lobby in Belfast, got the necessary forms signed and started on the course the following Monday.

The progress on the course was phenomenal and my outlook on life immediately changed. I felt like I had a purpose for living. The course ran from 9a.m. to 4p.m., Monday to Friday and I felt that I was living again. The interesting thing is that one month into the course I got a phonecall from the person in the government department that I had originally called. She told me that she had arranged a place on the course for me – the same course that I had already completed one month of. I laughed at the stupidity of the system and felt strangely satisfied at having made it happen against the odds, something I had always enjoyed previously.

The point of the above story is to explain how much we can achieve when we finally accept our reality and move on. If we understand the normal emotional stages that we go through, then we can look at our lives and see how we are dealing with our situations. In time, we pick up the skills to make the most of life. We must look at ourselves as objectively as possible and ask ourselves if we are living the life we want to live. I now realise the moments when I am in denial and I know how to deal with them. I sometimes catch myself wishing for some good luck or blaming someone else for my problems before realising that I must take responsibility for myself. In time, through my experiences, I have become more skilful at overcoming obstacles. Acceptance is the most important skill to learn. When we reach the point of acceptance we are ready to take the first step on our journey.

Main Points

- You must accept your current reality before you can take control of your life and change it for the better.
- It is easy to deny the truth of your situation and it might well make you feel better in the short term but in the long run it is damaging your chances of success.
- When you have examined your life and started to realise that it is not what you thought it was it is easy to blame other people but this won't do any good. The responsibility lies with you.
- There is little point in looking for miracles – it is better to decide to make your own luck.
- Take responsibility for your own life now and decide that you are going to achieve the success you want.

Try These Exercises

Exercise 1: Where am I?

Take a blank piece of paper and draw a line vertically down the middle of it. At the top of the left column write 'Great Things'.

Now think back over the last couple of years of the things that you wanted to do. Write down all of the things that you wanted to do both in your work time and leisure time and include both those you have done and haven't done. 'Great Things' can be learning the guitar or spending time with family or getting a promotion or anything else you want. Have fun with it.

Now in the second column write 'Real Things'. In this column write down the anatomy of one week in your life. Write down the activities that you have done in the last week, both good and bad. Now add some of the activities from six months and a year ago that you might have done in the course of a week.

Now cross out all of the items that appear in both columns. How many are crossed out in the 'Real Things' column? How many activities are you doing each week that really excite you? How much from the 'Real Things' column could you replace with things in the 'Great Things' column?

This should give you an idea of where you are and, more importantly, where you could be. Once you accept this, you are ready to set forth on the road to where you could be.

Exercise 2: Where did I go wrong?

Look at all of the activities that have not been crossed out in the 'Great Things' column from Exercise 1. Take each one in isolation and ask yourself why you haven't done this activity. Write down the reason on a piece of paper.

Does the reason survive scrutiny? Perhaps there is an element of denial or blame in there that stopped you from doing this activity. If it was on your list of 'Great Things' then it is obviously something that you think is valuable and will give you satisfaction.

Now ask yourself, what could I have done differently to have made this happen? How could I have taken responsibility? I guarantee you, the more times you do this, the more you will realise that you can control these activities and make them happen.

3

TAKING THE FIRST STEP

IN THE PREVIOUS CHAPTER I talked about finding the 'big red dot': the point you are at in your life right now. It involves taking a long hard look at yourself and getting to know who you are and where you stand in a world that is constantly changing. We cannot make time stand still, nor can we prevent the unexpected happening, but what we can do is accept what is going on in our lives and consciously take steps in the direction of where we want to go.

The stories throughout this chapter describe the challenges that people face when deciding what steps to take. Some involve major changes but there are also tales about the seemingly insignificant barriers that others have faced in their lives. Essentially what I am challenging you to do in this chapter is to decide whether *you* are going to choose the next steps in your life or let someone or something else dictate them to you.

This chapter is about taking the initial steps in the direction of the life that you really want.

Some people have very specific goals and know what they want to achieve far into the future but most people have little or no idea. If you are one of the latter, don't despair. As I have said before, many of the best journeys start with no particular destination in mind. It is worth putting some thought into the general direction, however, and starting the journey by simply taking the first small steps in that direction. Too often we look at the enormity of what we might like to do and never do anything about it. We forget that all it takes is one small step in that direction followed by another and before we know it we arrive at the destination. Take writing a book for example, it starts with one word, then a sentence, a chapter and ultimately a book. The book is the final product but the content of the book begins with writing just one word.

Taking the first steps can be difficult. When I took my initial steps after blindness, I had no idea what I could do with my life. I didn't have a clue what I wanted to do or even what a blind person was capable of. Those first steps after accepting that I had gone blind involved arming myself with the ammunition to create a future for myself. What that future would be, I didn't know, but the initial steps involved getting a stick, a guide dog and a computer with adaptive technology, and then learning to use them all. Walking the streets on my own, using a computer and reading my watch were all things that I had taken for granted before blindness and the last thing I wanted to do was learn them again. Instead, they were the first small and, at the time, irritating steps that I realised I had to take if I was going to approximate a life that I would have deemed successful by my pre-blindness definition. Small and insignificant steps maybe, but without them I would be doing none of the things that I now enjoy.

I had to swallow my pride. I accepted that I would have to go through the process of doing things that I really didn't want to do. I had to ask for help, listen to people that I didn't want to meet and face the fear of stepping into the world as a blind person. At the time it was terrifying but by facing my fears I soon ended up in a position where I was able to do things again. The problem was I wasn't quite sure what things I should do with my new skills. What would my future be? What would I do next?

Although I had taken the first steps towards a new life and was really already on a journey of sorts, at the time I did not sit down and write a list of goals and go after them. The process was emergent and involved a series of small steps moving me towards a destination that might seem quite simple to you: I wanted to live an independent life. An 'independent life' for me at the time meant being able to do the same things that I could do before I became blind. To achieve this aim you might expect that I designed a step-by step process that included goal-setting, planning and action, but truthfully I wasn't as organised as that.

I have read lots of books advocating goal-setting and ultimately achieving, but that was not what I did in the early days after blindness. As a result, I am not necessarily an advocate of it. I do not believe that goal-setting is applicable to all people at all times, although there is certainly a place for such an approach and I will explore that later in this book. During the initial phase of my rehabilitation I didn't know what my limits were and, as a result, could not set specific goals for my future. What I could do was take small steps towards some kind of future, even when I did not know what that future would be.

Sometimes when I am giving lectures I meet people who really want to make a change but don't know where to start. The most recent example of this is a guy I met in Singapore called Billy. He told me that he looks at people who are successful and thinks they have an aura about them that he does not have. I asked him what the difference between him and them is and he told me that the people he admired seemed to be much more focused than he is. He said he didn't even have any idea of what to focus on and added that he saw me as one of these focused types. It is true that I am now very focused on certain things but that wasn't always the case. I imagine few people set out on a career or life-plan knowing exactly how it will turn out. There was a long period where I felt completely lost and things only changed for me when I started concentrating on things that I like and things that interest me. I think that if you want to enjoy things then you should do things that you enjoy and if you want to be interested by the things that you do then you should do things that interest you. It might sound simple, but there are more people who don't follow this policy than people who do.

Do what you like, like what you do

There are many people out there who have no idea what they want to do. If you are one of these people, perhaps the first question you might ask yourself is: 'what do I like?'

I am not talking about what you specifically like to do every minute of every day but rather what do you enjoy doing at a very broad level? I enjoy travelling, sport, socialising, spending money, competition and understanding human behaviour. All of the things that I am now doing are in some way related to those broad areas of enjoyment. My work, sporting adventures, friends and academic research are all geared to satisfying those aims. Six years ago I didn't know what I would be doing to achieve these aims, but by doing things that moved me towards these broad interests I find myself in a position of incorporating them into my work. The hardest part was taking the initial steps and getting past the things that potentially were going to stop me achieving what I now am living.

For a time I wanted to be an investment banker because I

thought that would be something that would garner the respect of my peers and make me rich and powerful. When I lost my sight, the immediate opportunity to do that passed. Later, I thought about moving back into that area and becoming an economist but I figured out that this simply didn't interest me. There are many instances in my life where I have done things for the wrong reasons. Inevitably they have turned out to be things that in time I have realised I don't like and don't really want to do.

In the simplest form, what I do enjoy and what I am interested in is sport, interacting with people and running a business. I love doing these things and they form the basis of my career and of my entire life. Still, it took me a long time to discover this. Having lost my sight, it was only after I started rowing again, did a business master's and began to socialise, that I saw the possibilities that existed if I just pursued my interests. If you want to like what you do then do what you like.

There's a game you can play that will help you to understand what I mean. Look at some of the people that you know and consider whether you think they are successful and happy or not. Then look at their personality and interests. See if the people who are doing jobs that suit their personalities are the people who are successful and happy. I bet they are! I'll give you a couple of examples. I have a friend who loves sport and is incredibly knowledgeable about the history of all sports. He has a voracious appetite for all literature related to sport and as well as this he is brilliant with words. Every time he sends me an email I am in awe of his wizardry with words. He could make you laugh or cry with the turn of a phrase. Guess what job he does? He's a lawyer and he hates it. That's not because there is anything wrong with being a lawyer, it's because this guy was born to be a sports writer and he became a lawyer because it was a family tradition. In contrast, I know another fellow who is also fantastic with words and loves to argue. He is a brilliant speaker, interested in politics and fascinated by the notion of justice. Guess what job he does? He's a lawyer, and he loves it.

Follow your Strengths

I will stay in the area of law for the next person that I want to discuss. I have just spoken about the importance of following things that you are interested in. Another approach can be to follow things that you are good at. These two things are not mutually exclusive because the best situations will involve doing things that you love and are also good at. Jennifer is a good example of a person who has used both of these approaches in her life.

When she was in school she always liked art and she was good at it. She naturally followed her interests from a young age and decided to become a graphic designer. She completed her design studies and became a graphic designer, rose through the ranks and became successful very quickly. She enjoyed her job but soon realised that she was also interested in law and decided to study it in her spare time. She did not necessarily expect to practise as a solicitor and initially took on a four-year programme of study more out of interest rather than as a specific career goal. A few years on she is now a solicitor and has left graphic design in the background. In both spheres she was very happy in her career and has done well. When we asked her about the path she has taken, everything seemed so natural to her. She took each step forward based on what she liked and what she was good at. Many of us who are unsure of what steps to take would be well advised to do the same.

In the course of writing this book we also met John, who works for Cultivate, the sustainable living and learning centre in Temple Bar in Dublin. John's path has taken him to a point where he is doing something that he is not just interested in but that he also believes in. It is another thing to consider when you are wondering what path to take in your life. What do you believe in? John worked in advertising in San Francisco, a job that seems very far from what he is doing now. The journey is an interesting one. John originally completed a degree in property economics and a postgraduate diploma in business studies before moving to the United States to work.

To give you an idea of the kind of person John is, it is worth hearing a story from his college years:

I chose property economics because I thought it would be a good course. And it was. I felt it would be a good all round business degree to do. It seemed to have a little bit of everything. And it was very good on understanding investment. It also had a little bit of urban sociology in it; a little bit of the humanities to some extent. I liked that part about it. It even had a little bit of law, a lot of law actually. So it was quite rounded. But I didn't really know what university was all about. If I knew then what I know now, I probably would have done something more like arts, or something like English; something a little bit more creative. So, when I finished it, I was a bit disappointed. In fact when they asked, 'how would you change this course?' the thing that I said was that I would do more English literature in it. Because, I said, the problem with the course is that you are graduating people who are defining or analysing the world based on a year's purchase, on yield. If it makes sense from a yield point of view to kick the grannies out of the flat then that's what we'll do. I thought they should integrate a bit of emotion in to the course. Apart from that, it was grand. I got the degree and off I went. I still didn't know what I wanted to do at that stage, so I did property economics for a while.

Despite his doubts about the morality of property economics, John worked for a time in Chicago as a property appraiser for an estate agent before moving west to San Francisco. He worked there for an advertising agency and spent six years as an account manager for pharmaceutical and biotechnology companies. After a while he began to question the fact that he was using his talents to sell products. Over time he felt that the pharmaceutical companies were more interested in making profits than in healing people.

John wasn't sure what the next step should be, so he decided to explore. He went travelling in Europe and visited Holland, Germany, Poland, Romania and the Czech Republic. He was seeking inspiration for his next step. Something might hit him while he was away, he thought, something like buying a bar in Romania or opening up a hostel in Poland. He returned to Dublin and considered various business ideas, and thought briefly about importing log cabins from Norway and launching Ireland's first advertising blimp. However, he couldn't really muster the necessary passion for any of these things. John wanted to find something that he could really believe in.

Cultivate organises the Convergence festival every year. It promotes the idea of a new cultural wisdom that recognises and values the balanced, interconnected and holistic relationship between society, the economy and the environment. John volunteered for the festival and found that he believed in the idea of restoring a balance to society. He also felt that he had a contribution to make. After the festival he became more and more involved and is now in charge of communications at Cultivate. Although he is making far less money than he did when he was an account manager in San Francisco, he admits that he is happier now. He might later move on to starting a related business and who knows what he might yet achieve. Still, he is more than satisfied with his journey at the moment. Volunteering for the Convergence festival was the first step that took John on a journey he believes in.

Be Prepared to Try

By trying new things you are challenging yourself. You are seeing what you are capable of and finding out what you like. You might find a job that you like, or love. You might find an occupation that you believe in and gives you great satisfaction. That's what happened to John. He was prepared to get out of his comfort zone and look around for inspiration to help him take a step towards a different life. When you have come up with an idea of some of the things that you might like to do it is sometimes hard to take that first step. One of the best ways to take things forward is to give things a try. If there is something that you like, or you think that you could be good at, then give it a try. There are plenty of opportunities out there for attempting something, like taking a course or volunteering for a position. If you think that you might like to be a teacher, for instance, why not volunteer to help kids with their homework at a local community centre? There is very little to lose in giving something a try.

While researching this book we interviewed a guy called Paddy who, like many people, had no idea what he wanted to do. He grew up as the middle child in a large, quite conservative, family. His father was a policeman and most of his siblings ended up working in 'safe' jobs. While the rest of his family were quite reserved, Paddy was always a performer. He was a 'messer' and a clown and most certainly the odd one out in his family. He told us that as a child he considered himself more his father's suspect than his son. He didn't do particularly well in school and made it into a small college on the back of one of his brothers having done well there. Eventually he got a job as an office junior in a freight company.

His company offered to train him as an accountant and he accepted. Really he decided to do it because his girlfriend was a trainee accountant and it meant he would be able to spend more time with her. He qualified as an accountant and got a job with Bic, who make pens and women's hosiery. Later he moved to EMI, the music company, as a credit controller. The job suited him well. He set up a credit control system that worked like clockwork and he spent his time meeting clients for coffee or lunch and collecting cheques. For an outgoing person, it was an easy job.

Halfway through his stint at EMI, Paddy bumped into an old school friend who was doing comedy in the International Bar in Dublin. Some comedians had set up a club called the Comedy Cellar and Paddy went along to see what it was like. In his own words, he was blown away. He was addicted. He loved it. It took two years before he stepped onto the stage and tried it for himself. He wanted to do it, but it took him a long time to actually make the leap. When Paddy first got on stage he did a five-minute set and he brought the house down. Two weeks later he did a ten-minute set and it didn't go so well. Paddy recalls:

The place was packed for my first gig. 'Good evening Ladies and Gentlemen. It's the Comedy Cellar's tradition to have a new comic first on after the break. Please welcome Paddy Courtney.' I arrived on stage and whatever drug or drink or anything I've ever taken in my life could never match the elation of standing there performing to a group of people who have paid money to be made laugh. I was constantly at the top of the rollercoaster waiting to drop. That was the feeling, as if I had taken in breath but couldn't breathe out. It was an amazing feeling. I thought, 'Oh my God, I've found it. This is what I want to do. I want to entertain.'

Two weeks later they gave me another slot and this time it was ten minutes long. I thought it would be easy, I was able to do five minutes in my sleep the last time. I learned the ten minutes off by heart and said it in the mirror about forty times between the first gig and the second one. I was so blasé about the whole thing that I took pauses to let the audience's laughter die down while I was practising in front of the mirror. I was thinking, 'they'll easily be laughing for thirty seconds at that one, because that's a killer line.' I arrived at the gig and got up on stage. First gag, nothing. Second gag, nothing. By the third gag my nerves started kicking in and my voice began to wobble. I could see a girl at the back of the room folding her arms and I could lip-read what she was saying: 'this guy is shit.' I took a deep breath, did the entire ten-minute set in about three minutes. I didn't wait to get paid, I didn't wait for anything, I just ran out and I said to myself, 'who do you think you are fooling, you idiot?'

Eventually, after ten months on the sidelines, Paddy got on stage again and he still does it. Now he's no longer an accountant, he's a successful comedian and loves what he does. For years he had just gone with the flow and then he found something that he liked. Despite the early setback he knew that being a comedian was the thing that he wanted to do. It was inevitable that he would find his way back to it. One of the important things to note in Paddy's story is that he was prepared to give comedy a try. Although it isn't easy to get on stage in front of a crowded room, he really had very little to lose. After all, he had a well-paid and secure day job and he could always return to that. Being prepared to try things is an important part of finding things that interest you. Trying a new direction doesn't have to be risky. Paddy used his spare time to follow his comedy interests and it eventually led to him finding a new career that he loves.

Ruth was another person who didn't know what she wanted to do. She applied for a communications course when she was in school but wasn't accepted. She ended up studying European studies and all thoughts of communications went out of her head. While she was in college, she had little notion of what she wanted to do afterwards. When the college radio station was looking for presenters for 'rag-week', a friend persuaded her to go along to a meeting. Ruth was the only female to show up and because the ruling body, the IRTC, insisted that a certain percentage of radio presenters must be female, she was in high demand. Offered several hours of presenting a day, she was a little concerned by the fact that she only owned three CDs. Ruth is naturally quite shy so it took a little bit of persuasion before she finally agreed to do it. Sure I'll give it a try, she thought to herself.

She arrived for the breakfast show on the first day and was shown how to turn the microphone on. 'You start in five minutes,' she was told. 'I learned at that moment that my nervous reaction is a terrible feeling of nausea in my stomach,' she told us. After ten minutes, however, she felt quite comfortable. Ten minutes after that, the station manager came in and said, 'Wow, you sound like Dave Fanning!' Was that a good thing because she sounded like a top DJ or a bad thing because she sounded like a guy, she remembers thinking. Regardless, she loved it. She was hooked. When other people didn't turn up to present their shows, she happily replaced them. Students in Limerick were treated to ten hours of the Ruth show! After that week she sent in a tape to a 'DJ for a Day' competition being run by *Hot Press* and 2FM. She made the final but didn't win, but she knew now that this was what she wanted to do.

From there she began to do a weekly show on student radio. In addition, she rang all of the radio stations in her area and was given bits and pieces of work with them. Once she knew what she wanted to do, she chased it with enthusiasm. The following year she won the 'DJ for a Day' competition and was offered a job doing the traffic reports on the national broadcaster RTÉ. Next she went on to do the breakfast show on a new local station in Limerick, before being offered a job back in RTÉ doing various shows. When we spoke to her she was the breakfast presenter on 98FM, the most important position of the day at Dublin's biggest commercial radio station. Since then she has gone on to do the breakfast show on national radio. On the airwaves, it's one of the best jobs you can get. She gave radio a try and she hasn't looked back since.

Take the First Step Now

Like Ruth, I didn't know what I was going to do next. One thing I did know is that I had to do something. I knew the world was not going to stop for me and I couldn't sit in my bedroom for the rest of my life. I wanted a job. The desire to work wasn't even driven by the necessity to earn money, but rather it was the fact that I was supposed to be working and the fact that I would have been working if I hadn't lost my sight. Many of my friends had started jobs and it seemed somewhat attractive to be wearing a suit and earning my own money. I did this first in a plc in Ireland called IAWS Group and later in a business consultancy start-up that eventually went bust. Neither of the jobs I did were exactly the same as the finance job that I had sought in university but they did satisfy my need to work. In effect, I proved that I could be like my peers and gain employment.

Taking that first step was incredibly difficult. I didn't know if I could really do a job effectively, in fact I didn't even know if I would be able to get from my apartment to the job on time to start work. I didn't know the answers to lots of these questions but the fears I had were nothing compared to what I would be doing if I did not confront them. My fears about stepping into the world as an independent person away from the safe environment of my family were huge but the prospect of drifting through life in an insulated world was worse. In the same way, it was inevitable that Paddy would become a comedian once he had discovered it because it was much more attractive to him than being an accountant. That didn't make the first step easy. It still took him two years and a lot of soul-searching to make the step but rarely do we lose out when we take that step. Rarely do we suffer when we give something a try. Often our only regret will be that we didn't do it sooner.

When I completed my computer course I was conscious that I wanted a job but after conversations with a number of different employers it was evident that they didn't know if I could do a job as a blind person. And perhaps more importantly, I too was unsure of my capabilities and was not confident enough to really sell myself to an employer. The result was a lot of interesting conversations over cups of coffee in boardrooms, but no job offers. If I didn't believe in myself, I could not really expect companies to believe in me.

It wasn't until I was given a break that I was able to take that step. Until then, I was stuck at the start of my journey as a blind person with mobility and computer skills who was willing to start a job but didn't really know what he was capable of. IAWS Group plc, an agri-food business in Ireland, gave me that break and in particular Philip Lynch, the managing director of the company, identified my desire to work and allowed me to 'have a go'. With the understanding that I could not be sure that I would be able to do everything they asked of me but that I would try my best, the company and its employees were willing to start a journey in the workplace with me. I didn't know where it would end up and neither did they but we were both willing to take the first step, and the second and so on. Philip Lynch realised that although we weren't sure of my destination within the company, I could at least contribute something while taking the journey.

When a person receives a 'break' like I did, it is important to take it. I used my time in IAWS to develop my computer skills, my mobility and my ability to survive in the workplace and interact with people in a business context. I explored different areas of the business from event management to treasury reporting, some mergers-and-acquisitions work, waste management procedure and finally a fledgling e-commerce strategy. By facilitating my move into the workplace and assisting with my personal development, IAWS Group helped me to satisfy my desire to work in a job with status similar to the investment-banking job that I had originally hoped to do. By taking the first steps I was finding out about myself and what I was capable of and building my skills and confidence. It will be the same for you.

Next, I moved to an e-commerce business and technology

consultancy at the height of the dot-com bubble in early 2000. But during my time in the consultancy I increasingly felt under-qualified because almost everyone in the organisation had some kind of master's degree and I hadn't even sat my final exams in Trinity, although they did award me my degree based on work to date. I applied to a leading business school in Ireland, the Michael Smurfit Graduate School of Business; the course was a master's in business studies specialising in e-commerce. I didn't think I would necessarily get a place but I approached the application process in a way that I would appear to be as qualified as anyone. In an effort to bolster my chances, I demonstrated my interest in the subject by getting involved with e-commerce start-up networking groups, developing a business plan for my own e-commerce business, met with the course co-ordinator to discuss the content of the course and asked a PR expert to edit my application form. If I was going to do this, then I was going to show enthusiasm and really give it my best shot.

My application was successful. The thrill of gaining entry to such a course at the height of the e-commerce boom was extremely satisfying. I felt I was almost back to my pre-blindness self. I had put myself on the line by applying for something that I was not confident I had the ability to complete. I applied for a part-time place that would allow me to mix college with a full-time job. I performed better in those exams than any other set of exams I had ever done. I was not and am still not an academic but I was willing to have a go. The funny thing was that as soon as I got accepted and as soon as I started on the course the mystery of doing a master's was gone and as a result the fear of failure also disappeared. I was worried that I wouldn't be able for the master's, but it turned out to be fine. It is so often the case that our fears are misplaced.

I would like to add to this that there are applications of these ideas to business too. When I give talks, the same comment comes up in lots of companies. Often people in organisations are unwilling to try something new because they have operated in a company that has, in the past, not facilitated that freedom. Sometimes in the past if they were to take a first step they would have been castigated, and then a new regime comes in and expects or hopes that they will start to innovate! I am of the opinion that seven of the most dangerous words in businesses are: 'we have always done it that way.' There is always room for companies to try new things and for them to encourage their staff to do the same. Both in business and in our lives, taking the first steps can be difficult but if we don't take the first steps then we are going nowhere.

*

In this chapter I have outlined the first steps that I took. My story might well be different to yours. I had no idea what my first steps should be but getting a job, any job, was a huge step for me. You might already be in a job, but you might not know what the first step is to a new job. You might want to figure out the first step to a promotion. The truth is that we take the first step over and over again in life. Although we might not be sure of the final destination, we can at least take control of the direction we are taking. The key to making the right first step is to look at yourself and think about what your preferences are. Each person is different to the next. If we follow the things we enjoy, that we are good at, and that we believe in, we will rarely stray from a good path.

There are few things in life that aren't done better when they are done with enthusiasm. If you are looking for the first step, then search with enthusiasm. If you are trying something new, then attempt it with enthusiasm. And if somebody gives you an unexpected chance, then grasp it with enthusiasm. Paddy, John and Ruth all gave something a try and then followed it with enthusiasm. They found things that they thought they might like and did them despite being nervous or fearful. It can't be an easy thing to get up on stage to do comedy, to present a radio show, or to leave a well-paid job in California, but there is something more satisfying about doing the thing you enjoy.

My own experiences of taking the first step have taught me that on almost every occasion it is more difficult in theory than it is in practice. As unlikely as it might sound now, I have always had the option of going home and having my family look after their blind son. There were times when I felt that I would never be able to do any of the things that I wanted to. There were a few mad moments when I was lying face down on my bed, my pillow soaked with tears, that I feared my life was over. As I began to take small steps, as I began to try things that I liked, I found that this fear was misplaced. I began to find things that I liked doing and, because of the difficulties I had, I embraced them with the enthusiasm of a father who is welcoming back a prodigal son.

Taking the first step is never easy, but neither is it as difficult as it seems prior to taking it and, when you take the first step, all of the subsequent steps become easier. So, take those first steps now and start a journey that will take you in the direction that you want to go.

Main Points

- Once you have accepted the truth of where you are, you are ready to take the steps towards where you want to be.
- Knowing which direction to take is not easy, but a good start is to do things that you like and that you are good at.
- If you pursue things that you like and things that you are interested in then you are likely to enjoy what you do and be interested by them.
- Don't be afraid to try things – you have nothing to lose but the life you don't want.
- There is nothing to lose in trying things you have never considered before.
- Take the first step now, the only thing that you might regret is not having done it sooner.

Try These Exercises

Exercise 1: Charting my Steps

Take a blank piece of paper and write at the bottom something you love to do that took you time to learn. Perhaps it is ice skating, or maybe it is playing cards. At the top of the page write 'Before' to signify a time when you had never done this activity. What was the first step you took? And the second? Write down every step that took you from 'Before' to the point where you now do and enjoy this activity. This will illustrate to you how many steps we go through to end up doing things that we like. If you love swimming, perhaps the first step was finding your local pool. There might even have been a step before that where you asked a friend where the local pool was located. Steps in between might include finding the time to do it and taking lessons to improve. No matter the activity and no matter how good we become at it we had to take a first step at some point. Even the world's greatest golfers missed the ball with their first swipe.

Exercise 2: Learning to Try

In the exercise in Chapter 2 you wrote down a list of 'Great Things' – these are both things that you would love to try and those you love to do. If you didn't make a list then make one now. Have you tried any of the new things? Why not? Make a plan to try one of them in the next week. If you like the activity, keep doing it. If you don't, then go back to your list and try another. The more new things you try, the more natural it becomes to try new things, and the more things you find that you like doing.

4

MAKE IT HAPPEN

I HOLD THE VIEW that there are two types of people in the world and this observation has probably been the main driving force behind writing this book. As I see it, there are some people who mainly 'make it happen' and there are others who mainly 'make excuses'. I say 'mainly' for both because making it happen and making excuses define people at the extremes of a spectrum. At one end of the spectrum are people who seem to never do anything productive and instead put their energy into coming up with excuses and explanations for why they never get anything done. I'm sure you've met people like that and I have certainly met many. However, I have also met people who seem to never make excuses, but instead make things happen. Which end of the spectrum would you rather be on?

Excuses and Regrets

Let me explain what I mean by the type of person who mainly makes excuses. I am talking about people who, having faced up to the reality of what is going on in their lives as described in Chapter 2, then develop excuses that stop them really chasing what they want. We have all been one of these people at some stage in our lives. In the past I have at times wanted to do a certain thing but made excuses that have stopped me from doing it. Often, I have just forgotten about it but there have been other times that I have regretted not having pursued it. In general, I would have been much better off if I had ignored the excuses and just made it happen.

You might know that there is something that you want to do but still haven't done it. You might even regularly tell people that you would do a certain thing if you could. I've heard it so many times. 'I'd love to go back to college, but I just can't afford it,' says one person. 'I really want to train for a triathlon but I just haven't time,' says another. It sounds reasonable when people say that, but isn't it funny that other people go back to college and train for triathlons all the time? The difference is that some people make things happen and others make excuses. If we recognise that in ourselves and do something about it then we can achieve the things that we want to.

You might think that a chapter of this sort would be better positioned prior to the last one, which was about taking the first steps towards change. It's true that people often make excuses before they even consider doing something new; that is, before they even take the first steps. However, it is when people have decided what it is they want to do that the most damaging excuses kick in. Once you have decided on something that you would like to do or try, there is no reason not to do it. Excuses, at this point, are your enemy.

Take Paddy for example, after his second stand-up comedy gig his excuses took him off stage for several months before he got up there and started making it happen again. Paddy was no stranger to excuses at that time. He freely admits that before he found stand-up comedy he was free-wheeling through life, unsure of what to do and not even worrying about it. When he first observed the comedians in the 'Comedy Cellar' at the International Bar in Dublin he was blown away and it lit a fire in him. Despite this, it took him quite a while to give it a try. While he was saying to himself at the time, 'I want this, this is for me, I've got to try this', there was a feeling deep down that told him, 'no way, there's no way I'd stand up in front of people and do this'. It took him two years before he persuaded himself to finally do it. When he tried comedy, he loved it. The excuses that he had been making melted away. Since then Paddy has gone on to do numerous other things that would scare people. He specialises in warming up crowds before television shows, which is a tough thing to do. He has now started acting and was recently in an award-winning short film. He doesn't seem to make excuses anymore; he just goes ahead and does the things that he wants.

Another good example is Gavin who was also mentioned in earlier chapters. I admire Gavin very much for the way that he changed his career and pursued his dream despite the pressure on him not to change. Many people probably think he is crazy for having left a very secure and highly paid job to go back to school but he did it and is happy for having done it. Gavin will admit though, that it took him a long time to get to the point of making that decision. He made a lot of excuses despite the fact that he knew what he wanted to do. From the age of ten he knew that he wanted to be a doctor but he still made many excuses along the way and they almost prevented him from doing it. If they had, he wouldn't be as happy as he is now, having made the change. At some point the desire to become a doctor overcame the excuses and Gavin made it happen.

People who make it happen have few regrets. If you were to ask Paddy or Gavin what their regrets are in relation to becoming a comedian or a doctor it is likely that they would tell you that their only regret is that they didn't do it sooner. Those who make excuses often have many regrets. The number of excuses that you make regularly matches the number of regrets you have in life.

Stop Making Excuses

Making excuses is not unique to individuals; it happens in teams and companies too. I am talking now about the type of people, groups and organisations who have an idea of what they might like to happen, and for a moment even see the method by which they might achieve it, but somewhere in the midst of all that manage to come up with enough excuses to convince themselves that it is not possible. I have concluded from talking to many people at different levels that often we fail in our aims because we look at the possible, mix it with excuses and, hey presto, we've created something that is impossible. By deciding to take the excuses out of the equation we return the impossible to the possible. All it takes is a decision to make it happen.

I have been an excuse-maker in the past and sometimes I still make excuses but I am doing it less and less. There is a particular event in my recovery after losing my sight that illustrates in large part how I learned to stop making excuses. In 2001, three years after I lost my sight, things were starting to get back to normal for me. I had made it through the first steps and had become better at making things happen. I had a developing career, a place on a master's degree, and a life, but there was one notable gap and that was sport. Rowing had been central to my life before I lost my sight. It was a big part of my identity and much of the fun in my life; many of the friends and a lot of the motivation in my life was linked in one way or another to rowing. Despite the fact that rowing had been so much a part of who I was, it was the final thing I returned to.

For three long years, although I had a vague desire to return to the sport, I convinced myself that I had valid reasons not to get back in a boat. People would ask me questions like, 'are you still rowing?' and I would respond by listing reasons as to why I wasn't. The truth was that I wasn't in a boat because I simply hadn't made the concrete decision to do it. Despite the fact that I knew deep down I would love to be rowing again and benefiting from all the elements of it that I enjoyed before, I made excuses for not doing it. I told myself and the people who quizzed me that I didn't have time, that I was too tired after work, that I wouldn't be as good as before, that I didn't want to put myself through the hardship of training and racing anymore and so on. But all of these things were simply excuses that stopped me from doing what I loved to do – race boats.

In 2001, I decided to make rowing happen. I made the decision to get back into the boat and set myself the target of rowing for my country in the 2002 Commonwealth Regatta. The amazing thing is that as soon as I had made the decision to return to the sport, the excuses evaporated. I emailed a friend, Brendan Smyth, who I had raced with in university and told him that I wanted to see if we could qualify for the Northern Ireland team to go to the Commonwealth Regatta the following year. When Brendan arrived in April, we met up and started rowing. It was an uncharted route but we soon got the boat moving, linked up with a new coach, and slowly began getting fit. Before long we had secured two sponsors to fund our campaign and had won our trials and our first race in Belgium at the Ghent International Regatta. The season took off and later that year we went on to get silver and bronze medals at the Commonwealth Regatta in Nottingham.

I still talk to Brendan about the fact that the medals were really only a small part of the overall experience for me – the icing on the cake, if you like. For me, the training, the discipline and the friendships, in particular the bond that developed between Brendan and me, were almost more important than the medals. The sense of recovering an important part of my life, a thing that had been normality for me before, was vital. For three years I was out of a boat and it wasn't until I got training and racing again that I began to feel like a normal person; that is, to feel like the pre-blind Mark. The cumulative effect was massive. It was the last step of my rehabilitation from blindness and everything else since has been less about the blindness and more about the normal life choices that I would have made, blind or not. Leaving the excuses behind changed my life.

It all started with that simple decision. I said to myself, 'I am going to start rowing again.' The details of how I did it and the specific goals that I was aiming for came later. The starting point was a decision to get in a boat and do whatever I had to do to make it happen. Up to that point I had been making excuses for not facing up to the fact that I was using my blindness as a crutch for not rowing. I was unwilling to make time to train because I thought I was too busy with my job and master's degree but I spent a lot of time at the weekends in bed with a hangover. I wasted a lot of time in work putting in hours in the office to 'look like I was working' despite the fact that many people in the consultancy were doing very little as no work was being sold. I wasted a lot of time that I could have been using in a positive way.

I believe that often, lack of time is actually lack of time

management. Sure, the rowing itself was hard and I didn't enjoy every early morning on the river in the middle of winter or the weekly testing on the rowing machines or losing over ten per cent of my body weight to race in the lightweight category. But the excuses that had stopped me from returning to rowing in previous years were not there this time. In their place was a decision to make it happen. There was enough time to do it all if I was willing to organise my life better and accept the help of others, especially Brendan.

I will talk more about the help of others in Chapter 7, which is about teams but, as with most of this book, in this chapter I am focusing on individuals. Without my own decision to get back in a boat it would not have mattered who I was racing with, being coached by or being sponsored by. Although these people were critically important in helping me to achieve my goals, without an initial decision by me, I never would have pulled on my rowing kit in the first place.

Perhaps you find yourself in a similar situation. Is there something that you know you want to do but have been holding back for some reason? Have you been making excuses? Have you said, 'I don't have the time', or 'I don't have the money', or 'I'm too tired', when people have asked you why you don't go ahead and do this thing that you are interested in? Perhaps the thing that you want to do is to learn to play guitar. If you feel you would like to learn guitar but have only ever come up with excuses, maybe you don't really want to do it. Or, maybe you should make a decision right now that you will make it happen. Without a decision by you to make it happen and confront the excuses, you will never learn guitar and you might not achieve your potential in other areas of your life either.

I know that some of the reasons that stopped me rowing for years were simply excuses. Those excuses might have been facts of sorts but they were facts which, once I decided to come up with a solution, a way of dealing with them, were not things that needed to stop me rowing. So many of the excuses in our lives that justify us not doing something are often just excuses that can be overcome if we approach them from a different angle or with a different attitude.

My sister, Emma, is a good example of someone who made it happen instead of making excuses. Having worked as airport ground staff in check-in, ticket-desk and business lounge supervisor roles she wanted a change. From what she tells me, she enjoyed the interaction with people in her various roles in the airport but wanted to move on because the anti-social hours, poor wages and excessive commuting expenses left her tired and broke. She understood that her strength lay in dealing with people and she wanted more regular hours and substantially more money. I remember at the time thinking that although she wanted a sales job her sights were particularly high. It struck me that she was only interested in jobs that promised a company car and pay that, from what I could tell, would at least triple her salary. She had no experience in selling and no reason to get one of those jobs. But she did. There were numerous valid reasons why she should not even apply for them but they didn't seem to hold her back. She applied to many of these lucrative sales jobs and eventually got one … one year on from her first applications.

I am not sure if I would have done what she did. I am not sure whether I would have taken such a bold step to make that happen and pursued my aim with such gusto. However, she got a job that paid her an amount that she was happy with, she loved the job and she has had lots of company cars since. In fact she has been headhunted twice since moving into sales and has now joined a huge multi-national which is investing in her as a person through training and giving her the responsibility that she desires. Emma did not have it all set up on a plate. She just decided to take responsibility for her future by deciding what she wanted and making it happen. Sure, she doubted herself, but she dealt with the doubts and excuses and has achieved her goal.

Another person that I admire for his attitude is a good friend called Johnny. He was as interested as I was in getting a job in an investment bank in London. He applied to them and didn't get a job on a graduate placement. I remember sitting with him and another friend, William, in a café in Dublin one afternoon. Johnny told us that he was going to London after his degree and that he was going to get a job in an investment bank there. William's response was: 'you can't do that. You can't just move to London with no job and expect to get one.' Really, William was saying that he was not willing to do it. Johnny borrowed money from the bank, left for London and went to every recruitment agency he could find and met as many human resource managers as he could. He had a job within his first week. Johnny's story is a classic example of attitude. Yes, he has excellent people skills and yes, he had a good education but those are taken for granted in the type of job he was going for. The difference between William and Johnny is that Johnny was willing to have a go, willing to take a chance and not willing to give in to the excuses that potentially would have kept him in Dublin doing things he didn't want to do.

Christina, like Emma, made quite a significant career change.

Like my sister, she really made it happen. Christina studied drama at college and went to New York afterwards where she worked in an administrative capacity for an arts organisation. After two years working in the United States she decided to return home to Ireland and do a course in set design. She knew that she wanted to do something creative and preferably with her hands. A few days before she returned to Ireland, her father died. Reggie, Christina's father, had been involved in the rag trade for years and had saved a lot of materials in his garage when manufacturing had moved to Asia. He had hoped one day to be able to use all of these materials again.

Of course, all of Christina's family were deeply affected by the passing of her father. But Christina realised that she could do something with Reggie's legacy. He had left all of these materials behind him and she decided to use them. Instead of pursuing a course in set design she took a short course in bag making and established her own label, which she called 'Reggie' after her father. Suddenly she was her own boss and was running a business despite the fact that she had never studied business or anything like that. There are many excuses that Christina could have made along the way. She could have used her father's death as an excuse for not moving on or used her inexperience as an excuse for not taking up a new challenge. She could have said, 'I would love to start a bag-making business, but I don't know how to make bags and I don't know how to run a business.' She didn't make any excuses; she just followed what she wanted to do and made it happen. It is early days yet, but Christina has been successful so far and she loves the adventure.

When I think of people like Emma, Johnny and Christina I begin to think that it is easy to do the things that you want. The truth is that it isn't. Like great footballers, or public speakers, or teachers, they make it look easy. What they are good at is avoiding excuses and instead concentrating on the thing that they want to achieve. When I look at my life in this context I can see instances where I made excuses, and you probably can too. If there is something out there that you want to do or try but aren't doing it, is it because you are making excuses? If you take away the excuses, what are you left with? You are left with a decision. Are you going to do this thing, or are you not? Are you going to become a comedian, a doctor, a salesman, a craftswoman or not? When you take away the excuses the decision becomes clear and most often you will do the things you want to do.

Taking Control

When I talk about excuses I am talking about the things that stop an individual, team or organisation from achieving the possible. Up until now we have been talking about obstacles that could be melted by ending our excuses. The problems were within the control of the individual and, by having the right attitude, they could concentrate on making it happen instead of making excuses. However, sometimes our obstacles can appear to be immovable. Some things are beyond our control. A recent attempt at clay pigeon shooting made this very clear to me. I can tell you, it's very hard to hit a target that you can't see. But just because something is beyond our control doesn't mean that we can use it as an excuse. There is always a way of taking control of our situation, removing the excuses, and getting on with making it happen.

Take Helen for example. She is now the magazine features editor in one of Ireland's national Sunday newspapers. She is focused, determined and seems to have an overall plan that she is executing with success. However, where she is now did not just happen on its own and although she is satisfied with her current position and plans for the future, her career has not always been plain sailing. In the past she made excuses that hampered her progress and these excuses were often prompted by things that were outside of her control. At the time the excuses seemed valid and in many ways they were. After all, what could she do about these things that were outside of her control? Well, there were things that she could do, and eventually she did them.

Helen is a very impressive person. She comes across as someone who has so much ability and such a good attitude that her life and career come easily to her. However, despite my impression of her, she maintains that it has never been easy. She says: 'For a long time I felt as though I was struggling. I was like a round peg in a square hole. It was always hit and miss, and most of the reasons for this were beyond my control which made the situation very stressful.'

Having studied English and drama at the University of London and the Central School of Drama, Helen got a job with a newspaper in Belfast and more recently Dublin. But after the initial excitement of her first jobs, she describes feeling as though she had begun to stagnate. 'The newspaper had undergone various changes with regard to staffing and design and the result was that it became increasingly difficult to work on topics that were of interest to me. The newspaper actually decreased in size and there was less space for the feature articles I enjoyed writing. I often found myself working on material that I had no interest in. As a reporter I had no real control over content and so I began to feel as though I was going nowhere.'

Helen lost motivation because she was not working on

projects that she was interested in and, worse still, had no control over the work that she was given. She could have done what so many people do – that is, she could have done nothing at all and just got on with her job although she was unhappy. I bet there are many people you know who can tell you everything that is wrong with their lives and identify the problems, even going as far as to bask in their awfulness, but still do nothing to overcome them. Helen could have said that she was not writing the stories that she wanted to because the structure of the newspaper was not right for her and that there was nothing she could do about it. She wasn't in a position to change the management of the newspaper, so what could she do?

The frustration became too much and she began a search for solutions to the problems. She stopped making excuses for her situation and took control. In the first instance she looked for a way out of the newspaper and into another job. In September 2003 she decided that she needed to find a new job so she applied everywhere but got a series of rejections. Suddenly she had the opportunity for many more excuses at her fingertips – she could have decided that she wasn't good enough, didn't have enough experience or skills. But she wasn't prepared to do that, so instead she looked for help. She took some media training and followed that by making contacts with individuals who could lobby on her behalf. The pieces of her career jigsaw were coming together and her confidence was increasing. She was beginning to feel in control and she was determined to keep the momentum going:

Throughout the period of retraining and thinking about my career I began to feel more in control of where I was going. I decided to work on projects that interested me outside of my regular working hours. I began to feel happier, more in control and as though I was actually doing something that mattered. Then I decided to go to Cuba for five weeks to work as a freelance journalist. I thought of the reasons why I might not do it – maybe I would lose my job in Dublin, maybe I would hate Cuba, maybe I would not sell my stories. All of these negative outcomes were possibilities but at the time it did not scare me and I was prepared to risk them coming true. I left for Cuba and spent five weeks working in Havana. The decision to go to Cuba was probably the best that I have ever made. I decided to do it at a time when I was feeling very disheartened and frustrated so I thought that the only way to make myself feel better was to take control of the situation in any way that I could. Working in Cuba was difficult because of the absence of free speech and the overarching government influence, but I had a great sense of personal exploration and achievement upon my return. I also realised that I could change my own situation if I put my mind to it.

On returning to the newspaper, Helen found that her performance at work was improved by her overall change in attitude. The fact was that she was now in control of her career and the odd frustrating piece of work in the paper could not change that fact. Later an opportunity came within the paper to move sideways and upwards and because she was performing well, the change was an obvious one. Once Helen took control of her career, everything else fell into place and the excuses fell away.

There will always be things that seem to be outside of our control, but for every seemingly immovable object, there is a clever plan for getting around it. And very often, attitude is the key.

Positive Attitude

It is my belief that what I have achieved is, more than anything else, a result of attitude and deciding to make it happen for myself rather than giving way to the excuses that would stop me. It is hard to admit to yourself that excuses that have governed parts of your life are just excuses, rather than life-stopping or deal-breaking facts.

Throughout my rehabilitation and beyond I have had to face up to things that I had plenty of reasons to avoid. I had lots of what seemed like strong arguments for not doing many things but often they were nothing more than excuses caused by a lack of confidence, feelings of uncertainty and the fear of failure. By taking an objective view of what we are trying to achieve we will ask ourselves: 'am I going to let those negative messages stop me achieving my goal or is the prize worth more than the not doing it?'

Recently I stood on a platform high on Auckland Harbour Bridge with a thick elastic band attached to my feet. The elastic was a bungee cord and I was about to dive into the abyss. Everything in my head was telling me not to do it: 'I mean, think about it Mark – diving off a bridge, over forty metres up, is not something you should do.' But I had taken the first steps to doing the bungee jump by buying the ticket and climbing the bridge to the platform and in 5, 4, 3, 2, 1 … I did it. In a split second I forgot the excuses and, as I flew through the air experiencing the rush of the jump, the excuses were far from my mind. By making it happen, by diving over the edge, I now own the experience. If I had listened to the excuses that told me that it was a ridiculous thing to do then I would not have that memory to enjoy.

Similarly, and more seriously, I could have decided to end

my life as I lay face down in my bedroom with my life in tatters. My tears were red with blood after the operations on my eyes and I was deflated by the knowledge that I would never see again. I could have crumbled and made excuses for the rest of my life for not doing the things I wanted to do. I could have used my blindness as an excuse for leaning on my family, friends and the state for support for the rest of my life. But that is not living, and making excuses for what we cannot do is not living either. I can tell you that I didn't want to leave my house, never mind step into the workplace, at a time when I wasn't sure what clothes I was wearing or if I would be able to make my way to the office at all. I didn't want to put myself on the line by applying to a master's programme that I didn't think I would be accepted for or complete. And I certainly did not feel I could re-enter rowing, a sport that prior to going blind had been such a large part of my life. I made excuses to avoid these things because I thought I might not be able to do them.

*

One thing is crystal clear to me. Not doing something because you are not sure if you will be able to do it is simply an excuse. We do not find out if we can do something by avoiding it. We do not achieve the things in life that we want to by saying how difficult it is going to be or that everything is not perfect. We do find out about ourselves and our ability to achieve ambitions by deciding to have a go, to make them happen or at least to try. Excuses are the enemy of achievement. They stop people from doing the things they want and they stop people from becoming happy and satisfied with their life.

Forget the excuses and make it happen.

Main Points

- Be someone who 'makes things happen', not someone who makes excuses.
- Too often we make possible things impossible by simply adding excuses.
- The number of excuses that we make often matches the number of regrets we have in life.
- One of the most common excuses we make is that we don't have time but often lack of time is actually lack of time management.
- Changing your attitude can change your life.
- Excuses are the enemy of achievement – forget the excuses and make it happen.

Try This Exercise

Exercise: Losing the Excuses

Write down as a heading on a piece of paper something you would really like to do but haven't managed to achieve yet.

Underneath that heading, write down all of the reasons why you haven't done it.

Now, think creatively. Go through each of the excuses one by one and figure out a clever way of overcoming the problem. We all have the creative ability to overcome our problems and by taking each excuse in isolation we can reduce their gravity.

The excuses will melt away and the impossible will become possible.

5

TO PERSIST OR TO CHANGE? THAT IS THE QUESTION

WHEN WE ARE ON any journey, we have the option to turn off the road. We can take a different route that will bring us to the same destination and we can also choose a road that will take us to a completely different place. Just because we have chosen a path does not necessarily mean that we must stick doggedly to it and, by the same token, just because there are intersections in the road doesn't mean we have to change our course.

The point is that whether you decide to persist with your course or change to another one, it is a choice. If you decide not to change that is a decision in itself. Deciding to persist or deciding to change direction, in keeping with the theme of this book, is within our own control, even if at times both of these things seem alien to us. No matter what position you are in right now, the reality is that you will face the choice to either persist or change many times along the journey through life. But the choices that present themselves are not to be feared and to understand that they exist will help alleviate any fear that may arise.

We all face the choice to persist or change time and time again throughout our lives. The choice can be as simple as whether to get up in the morning when the alarm clock goes off or as complex as starting a process to re-engineer an entire business or restructure an entire country. In the following pages we deal with the issue of the basic choice that we face at all times in our lives: either to persist with the status quo or to choose to change it. I am not suggesting that change is always necessary. After all, if it is working why change it? But in light of the fact that everything around us is always changing we must be aware that persistence is one option and choosing to change is another.

'What's next?'

Throughout the rehabilitation period after losing my sight I was ticking boxes on a list that represented my pre-blindness identity. These boxes included things like living alone, socialising and meeting girls, getting a job, doing a master's and competing in rowing. All of the things that I did were in some way related to who I was before I went blind. Perhaps I was living my life backwards rather than looking to the future or perhaps it was a necessary process. Whatever the psychology, four years after blindness I was back to the old Mark. By the time I raced my finals in the late summer of 2002 at the Commonwealth Regatta and at the same time handed in my master's thesis, I had re-established some sense of normality in my life.

Despite the veneer of normality, the strange thing about the following few months was that they were in some senses more difficult to deal with than the initial stages of sight-loss but the difficulties were less about blindness and more about life direction. I had to deal with the questions of 'What next?' 'What do I really want to do?' 'How will I do it?' 'Why do I want to do these things?' Up to this point the goals that I had set and achieved were about who I was, not what I would do with myself. Just after losing my sight, the decisions I made required more attitude than conscious thought and by most other people's definitions, the fact that I even got out of bed made me a success never mind achievements in rowing or employment. But life does not stand still for anyone and while I did have a sense of satisfaction for making it back to 'normal', I didn't know what to do next.

I was faced with the difficulty of making some decisions. I had no job because the company I had been working for had folded, I had finished my master's and the rowing season was over. I had a blank slate to work from and it was awful! This may sound like the introduction to a chapter on goal-setting and planning but it is not. Prior to even thinking about the goals we set I think it is worth investigating the merits of both change and persistence. Both are issues common to us all and things that we can decide to do on many different levels.

Don't be Afraid to Change

First let me concentrate on change. For many of us change is difficult. If you walk away from something then you are often deemed a failure. If you change direction even after you have completed a project, often people around you question your motives. However, in my experience, change can be one of the most liberating experiences in life and deciding to change course or to stop what you are doing is not a failure at all.

I approach this subject as a person who does not like to 'give up'. I like to approach things with a mind to make them happen despite the difficulties, obstacles, barriers or excuses. I like to go after what matters to me and if somebody tells me that I can't achieve something it makes me even more determined. This is why I find this kind of change so difficult and why, I believe, it should be considered seriously in this discussion.

In September 2002, having been through a four-year process of rehabilitation, I was suddenly struck with the myriad of career options that faced me. I thought about applying to a management consultancy in a similar role to the one I had been doing in the company that had just gone bust but I didn't want to go back to that kind of working environment. At the start of an academic cycle I could have gone back to full-time education and I remember waking in the middle of the night to phone my dad to tell him that I was going to apply to become a barrister. In the middle of the night I was convinced that it was the career for me but it didn't make as much sense after sleeping on it. And so I returned to the idea of becoming an investment banker of some description. At the time, I was twenty-six years of age and thought that I might be in a stronger position to avoid the work that I hated in the consultancy, namely the work that new recruits get, if I was further educated in a relevant discipline. I researched what I might go into and convinced myself that becoming a trained economist would allow me to satisfy my desire to work in a cool job, earning lots of money in a role somewhere above entry level.

The goal was clear to me and I actually convinced myself that I would really fit the role. I saw myself on Bloomberg TV or Reuters commenting on the state of the world economy and writing expert opinion pieces in the *Financial Times* and *Economist*. I think that would still be an attractive proposition. The only trouble was that after researching a number of routes to achieve that goal, I started to realise that I had no interest in learning about the statistics, the econometrics and the other nuts and bolts of economics. The reality was that I would have to spend a year completing preparatory courses to be accepted into an economic master's which, in my plan, would allow me to do an economics PhD which would facilitate my ultimate aim of becoming a well-paid economics expert.

I began in Trinity College Dublin doing a diploma in statistics with some quantitative economics courses in October 2002. I went through the process of getting a large volume of material scanned into a special format so that my computer could read it to me and organising a reader to read some other material to me as well as to take notes in some of the more complicated classes. Yes, I was all set to go, but then I realised that I had little or no interest in the subject. It rapidly became clear to me that I was not going to be the next Alan Greenspan. I remember sleeping in my statistics lectures for the first couple of months and drifting in and out of consciousness in econometrics and economic theory. In fact, several snoozes later, it became clear to me that high level economics was not for me.

But I had committed to economics. I had told lots of people that I was going to become an economist. I had worked with the disability services in the university to access material and lecturers had gone out of their way to make it as easy as possible for me to do their courses. The idea of walking away from the plan before it had even got off the ground was my worst nightmare. I mean, I did not see myself as a quitter and that is what I thought I would be doing if I walked away from economics. I saw it as failure and I did not want to be a failure.

Around the same time I met a couple of fantastically interesting people who seemed to really enjoy what they were doing in life. One was Caroline Casey, who is visually impaired, and the other was Miles Hilton-Barber, who is blind. Miles and Caroline were then on the Irish leg of a trip that took them around the world using eighty forms of transport to raise awareness of the abilities of disabled people. When I met them for dinner, I noticed that the overwhelming enthusiasm they had for what they were doing with their lives was infectious.

By the time I met Caroline, Miles and the rest of the 'Around the World in Eighty Ways' team, I had already heard of Caroline. When I did my master's degree I had heard of a visually impaired girl who had completed another course in the university and come first in her class. That was Caroline. Subsequent to that, in August 2002, I heard her on the radio talking about disabled people in the workplace. At the same time I had been on the radio talking about my experiences as a blind person preparing for the Commonwealth Regatta with my rowing partner, Brendan. A number of blind people, or people with failing sight, contacted me after the show and it struck me that maybe in some small way I could do something to help. It was then that I made contact with her charity.

Caroline was born legally blind and had worked with Andersen Consulting, now called Accenture, for a number of years. In some ways I think she was trying to prove that her sight problem would not hold her back but my understanding is that she wasn't happy and became disillusioned with her job. It was at this point that she decided to do something that mattered to her and set about putting together a plan that would see her trek over 1,000km on a solo elephant-back voyage across India. She set up the Aisling Foundation in June 2000, as a registered holding charity for the Indian challenge 'to inspire people into thinking of disability in a positive way'. She was willing to change after a long period of worrying about leaving Andersens. She says that it just felt right and she now loves what she is doing.

I have a lot of admiration for the things that Caroline did

and still does but it was Miles who was pursuing the things that I could see myself doing. Miles has been blind for over twenty-five years. Originally from South Africa, he worked for many years in the Royal National Institute for the Blind in a role that involved giving advice to blind and partially sighted people on their career options and future direction. Later, he saw an opportunity to help educate companies and encourage them to create opportunities for the blind people he once advised. In this capacity he used his experiences to inspire individuals and teams but also to raise awareness of the abilities of blind people in the workplace. He continues to do that but now works for himself using his adventures to illustrate his presentations. During dinner I had a long chat with Miles about his background and his life now. As far as I could see he took part in amazing sporting adventures around the world and drew on those experiences to help companies deal with challenges in their organisations. It struck me that he had an unbelievably interesting life. At the time, I was involved in something that I hated and Miles was doing something that he loved.

I didn't give it any more thought until I got a call from Shell Ireland who were looking for a motivational speaker for an internal training day in their Dublin office. The Aisling Foundation, Caroline Casey's charity, recommended me as she was travelling around the world with Miles at the time on another project. They thought that my coping with blindness coupled with my recent success in rowing would be interesting for the group. I think there were about eighty people in the room for that internal staff training day in Shell. I loved the buzz of the performance, speaking in front of a group of people and, judging by their feedback, they enjoyed what they heard. I enjoyed being in command of my subject, which is in stark contrast to the difficulties I had been experiencing with economics. And that enjoyment was complemented by a pay cheque for my trouble. I suddenly realised that I could do what Miles was doing, that I could use the abilities that I already possessed to carve out a career and do things that I really enjoyed.

Also presenting to the group that day was a man called Ian. We had a chat afterwards and I discussed with him my difficulties with economics and we also chatted about a book called *The Elephant and the Flea* by Charles Handy. I had not read the book, but I had heard Handy speaking on the radio and was aware of some of his ideas. Ian had read the book and promised to send me a copy. The basic message that Handy communicates is that we can either sell our time to large organisations for a price as he did when he worked for Shell or the other option is to look at our skills and sell them to different organisations as they require them. Handy does not argue that we must all leave our jobs but he does argue that there is little point doing something that does not interest you – whether that be in a large organisation or a small one. Why persist with something that does not make sense to you? Neither you, nor the organisation you work for, will benefit from lack of enthusiasm. Persist with it if you choose to. Tell someone, and try to change within the organisation. Or leave. But realise that the decisions are up to you.

Having delivered the talk to Shell, chatting to Caroline, Miles and Ian, and thinking about Handy's arguments, I stopped pretending that I was going to be an economist. The first thing I did was to stop feeling guilty for not going to my economics lectures. The second was to plan my new future. Although it was liberating, walking away from economics was desperately difficult. I had told lots of people what my plan was, I had committed to the course and the associated goals, and I had, in effect, committed to a life. I was, and am still, not the type of person who likes to just drop something or fail to complete it, but this was a time when I had to say to myself and many others that not only had I made the wrong decision but that I was going to walk away from it. At the time, before I took the decision, I felt like it would be a failure. However, the reality was that persisting with something that I really didn't want to do would have been a greater failure. To walk away, to admit that I would be better served by changing direction, was the success.

My friend James is someone who has been faced by these kinds of choices on a number of occasions. The year he left school, when he was just eighteen years old, he was given the opportunity to sail full-time in an attempt to qualify for the Olympics. He was faced with a choice between persisting with his education and changing direction entirely to reach for the stars in a sporting context. In the end he felt like this opportunity was too good to turn down and, while all of his friends went to college, he was sailing in regattas all over Europe. After one year of full-time sailing he decided to combine his sailing with university study and returned to college. He was able to study and sail successfully and things were going well. As the Atlanta Olympics approached in 1996, it became clear that he was not going to qualify and so James did not have to combine his commitments any more. Strangely, his academic study suffered. The time pressure of sailing and studying at the same time had made him a diligent student. Now that he had time to study, he wasn't able to do it as well. He passed his third year in college but he didn't get the grades necessary to proceed to the final year.

He went to see the careers officer in the university to discuss his options. He could repeat third year or he could leave college now with a pass degree; the career advisor recommended that he leave college. She felt he did not have the academic ability to get the 2.1 grade that he probably needed to bolster his academic record after his problems at the end of third year. Furthermore, his sailing coach urged him to come and join him in his burgeoning coaching business. James was faced with a difficult choice: should he make a change or should he persist? He decided at that point to persist. He wanted to complete his academic life on a successful note and prove the careers officer wrong. That was his goal and he achieved it.

When he completed his studies he decided to persist with his interest in sailing and coaching. Although a lot of his friends were moving on to more standard business graduate jobs like banking, accountancy and consultancy, James decided to get involved in a small business with his sailing coach. Some of his peers thought this wasn't a 'real job' in the way that their jobs might have been, but in fact he was applying all of the things he had learned in business school on a day-to-day basis. The business grew. It became well known in sailing circles, began to employ people and won awards. However, after a few years James became tired with the struggle of maintaining a small business with inconsistent cash-flow. Although the business was surviving, he didn't feel that he could take it any further. After a long time of persistance he decided it was time to change. There was a lot of pressure at the time. He felt a responsibility to his business partner, his employees and the bank, but after a lot of thought he decided it was time to change. It was the right decision for him.

Leaving the company was one of the most difficult decisions James has ever made. When one has invested so much time, energy and money into something there is a great temptation to persist with it. Sometimes, however, it is right to make a change. Making a change like this is not a failure as long as you have given it real thought and consideration. In fact, making the right change is a success. James could have persisted with a job that was making him unhappy in the end. This, of course, would not have been helping him, or the company. In this case, making a change was the right thing to do.

Persistence

Let me focus now on persistence in greater detail. It is clear to me that it is important to be open to change and that if I am doing something that does not make sense to me anymore that I should change. Change is not a failure and I will discuss the subsequent actions that I took since changing from economics in the next chapter. I am not afraid to try new things and to take the decision to go down a wrong road once or twice. At the same time, I also think that if you decide to go after things with no thought in mind of the final destination then you could be destined to a life of hopping from one career to another without truly getting your teeth into anything. Sometimes the right decision is to persist.

Very often I get asked in seminars, 'are you always motivated?' Of course, the answer is no. We are not robots, we are human beings and, whether we like it or not, life can be difficult. The sooner we realise that we will continue to face obstacles, hardships and challenges the better. Perhaps I am fatalistic but I am less and less surprised when I come up against problems in my life. The first question I ask is, 'what can we do about it?' I do moan, get annoyed and experience varying degrees of happiness, as does everyone, because that is the way life is. It is important to realise that when we are trying to achieve something in our lives, it will often not be easy.

I immediately think of Nelson Mandela when I think of the topic of persistence. Today we think of Mandela as a grey-haired super-human statesman. For all Mandela's talents, I think the most telling one was persistence and that is something that we can all attempt to emulate. In a context whereby 'No matter how high a black man advanced, he was still considered inferior to the lowest white man', Nelson Mandela set about changing the status quo, even though he knew his actions at the time against apartheid in South Africa would get him in trouble. His efforts resulted in his imprisonment for some twenty-seven years.

His years on the notorious Robben Island made Mandela a virtual stranger to his family, and he often wondered whether the struggle was worth it. His mother died while he was there and he was not allowed to attend the funeral. Imagine not being able to attend the funeral of your own mother. On the rare occasion that he was allowed family visitors, he was given only half an hour with them. Because of the restrictions on her movements, he did not see his second wife, Winnie, for two whole years during his incarceration, and his children were not allowed to visit him before the age of fifteen.

In the latter years of his imprisonment, as his legend grew, white politicians began to listen to his ideas for a fully democratic South Africa. They knew that history was not on their side and the country was becoming explosive. Eventually, amid great euphoria, Mandela was released in 1990, having spent twenty-seven years in jail. As everybody in the world must know, four years later, after the country's first non-racial elections, he was elected president of South Africa. I will not pretend to understand the complexities of the South African situation nor am I commenting on the actions of either side, but I will say that Nelson Mandela's story is a classic example of persistence. He is an incredible example of choosing to persist in extreme circumstances and eventually achieving a positive outcome. Luckily, however, most of us do not need to go to jail or struggle to change a nation in our lives but we do have our own battles to fight and choices to make.

When we were doing the research for this book we met a local businessman who is a great example of the power of persistence. Ger first had the idea for a healthy fast food restaurant when he was in university. He was a keen sportsman and he always found himself looking for something healthy to eat that he could consume in a hurry. For his final year thesis he wrote a business plan for a healthy fast food restaurant but when he finished college he didn't pursue it as a business. He left for the United States and got a job in a bar. For a couple of years in America he worked in bars and had a lot of fun. At the same time he was gaining experience in the catering and service industry and his idea for a healthy fast food café never left his mind. He would tell anyone that would listen about his idea for a business, but nobody offered to help him. He saw how well-run and efficient the cafés in the United States were compared to those he had seen at home in Ireland and he believed an opportunity was there to be taken.

He came back to Ireland at Christmas one year with his business plan and had no takers. People told him that he was too young and that he had no experience, which he didn't really at that time, at least in Ireland. He had no finance at any level and it was quite an expensive business to get into. So he had no finance, no experience and, being from Cork, he also had no networks in Dublin. Nobody would take the idea on, so he went back to the United States. Still he didn't give up on his idea. He came back again at Christmas the following year and gave it another try. This time he intended to make more of a go of it and he had enough money to keep him in Ireland for a few months. He went around meeting people and trying to attract investors and when he came across a group of entrepreneurs who had a very similar idea he decided to join them.

As time passed the fledgling business became messy. There were too many directors and they all had their own idea about what the business should look like. Directors began to leave the enterprise, but Ger persisted because he believed in the idea that he had first thought of years before in college. Now there are only two directors, and Ger is one of them. Their café, Nude, is one of the most recognisable and popular in Dublin. They have opened several outlets and are constantly growing. By persisting with an idea that he could have given up on many times, Ger is running the business that he wanted to from the start. In this case, persistence led to Ger being successful and happy.

To persist or to change is a choice that we regularly face as individuals, as part of a team or as an organisation. Often we decide to persist with something that we know is wrong for us and if we choose to do that then we must also be willing to put up with the consequences of that choice. We can choose to change if something is not working but we must be willing to face the fact that change is never easy, even if in the long run it makes a positive difference. Whether you decide to persist or change is based on the circumstances that you find yourself in but the most important thing to remember is that persistence and change are both choices that you can make. You are in control of that choice.

Forced Change

There is another scenario that exists and it is a scenario that I know quite a lot about. There are times in our lives when we are forced to change by circumstances beyond our control. There are times when it is impossible to persist with our lives in the way that we have been. In my case, when I lost my sight I was forced to change by circumstances that I had no control over. When this happens we are clearly not deciding to change. Nevertheless we can choose how we respond to this change. For a chief executive that might mean changing the way his/her company operates. There are times when new legislation can alter the face of a market completely and it is always the company that reacts best that wins in the new environment. These are companies that realise it is how we respond to enforced change that makes the difference. Your life might change tomorrow. You might lose your job, or your partner or you might receive a bad performance review.

The question is: how will you react to this change?

Let me tell you the story of what I think is the most amazing reaction to forced change I have ever heard. At a recent conference I had the pleasure of listening to Tim Waterstone, who is the founder of Waterstone's bookstores and the Daisy & Tom children's department stores, and also a former chairman of HMV Media Group plc. That last sentence will tell you what a successful businessman he is, but the story I want to tell you starts with a moment in his life that wasn't so successful.

Tim Waterstone joined WH Smith in the UK in 1973 and rose steadily through the ranks only to be sacked in 1982. There can be few greater forced change situations than being sacked. He could have responded in many different ways. He could have been devastated and he was, but next he took action that left the company that sacked him devastated. Instead of disappearing into the corporate wilderness, he founded Waterstone's booksellers with £6,000 from his redundancy money and £100,000 in venture capital. His first shop was on London's Old Brompton Road.

With an openly confessed vendetta, Waterstone's express aim was to take WH Smith on head to head and beat them at their own game. Waterstone's booksellers began appearing beside or opposite WH Smith stores all over the UK. In fact, as Waterstone recounted at the conference, if they could open stores opposite and beside WH Smith then they did.

Waterstone's reputation grew to become perhaps the best literary bookshop in the world and changed the face of British book retailing. Waterstone's was also one of the two or three largest and most successful venture capital entities of its time. Despite his original vendetta, he sold Waterstone's to his former bosses nine years later for £47m and in the process made himself and many others extremely wealthy.

However, there is a twist in the story. Waterstone had a mental block in relation to WH Smith and despite having made a fortune from the sale, he could not get the thought of his sacking out of his mind and had nightmares about his former boss owning his company. As a result, he bought the company back again together with EMI and Advent International in 1998 creating HMV Media Group, of which he became founder chairman. At that point, he told us, the dreams, or nightmares, of the past disappeared.

Tim Waterstone's response is a clear example of taking control and responding to forced change in a positive way. Please don't misunderstand me: I am not advocating that being motivated by a vendetta is necessarily a good thing. I am saying that we can either let forced change control us or we can take control of our response to that forced change. Tim Waterstone could have taken his £6,000 and disappeared but he refused to be dictated to. He couldn't undo his sacking but he could control his response to it.

I am a strong advocate of taking control of our own decisions and, by extension, our lives. I would argue that in almost all circumstances we can decide what to do next. We can decide to react positively or negatively and I think you will agree with me that there is little point in reacting negatively. You might not like the changes that are forced upon you but the decisions you make about what to do next are what count. I was not in control of losing my sight. It was a change that was forced upon me and it is definitely not something that I wanted to happen. I've realised with time that by reacting positively to this enforced change my life can be every bit as good as it was before, if not better. I was in control of the response and I might have chosen to spend the rest of my life being looked after by others but instead I chose to take control and make the most of things. There is no reason why anyone else couldn't do the same.

We are not helpless passengers on a bus that is driving through our lives. You are in the driving seat and it is up to you to decide the route that you want to take. Of course, you might be sharing the journey with others and you might have to take their wishes on board, but that is your choice. On this road-trip you will have the opportunity to turn off, whether you change your course or stay on course is up to you. You might hit a dead-end from time to time and you will have to decide then what to do. In each of these cases the steering wheel is in your hands and you can decide where to go.

Main Points

- Whether you decide to persist or to change direction, it is a choice you are in control of.
- The choice of whether to persist or to change is one that recurs throughout our lives.
- Deciding to change direction does not necessarily mean that you are giving up. Don't be afraid to change.
- Obstacles and difficulties are inevitable in life and at times it is crucial to persist to ensure success.
- Don't make changes just because you find something difficult. If you really want to do something then persist. If you discover that you don't believe in what you are doing then the time has come to change.

Try This Exercise

Exercise 1: Persistence

A simple exercise to do here is to write down all of the things that you do in a week. All of them. It seems like a silly and tedious thing to do, but how often have you looked at your life in this detail. It's your life, if you don't look after it, nobody will.

Look at all of the things you are doing and ask yourself, 'why do I do this thing?' If you are unsure then put a question mark beside it. Take a closer look at all of those question marks and ask yourself why you are persisting with them. Do you have a good reason? If not, then perhaps it is time to stop persisting with this thing and change it.

6

'WHAT' AND 'HOW' BUT MOST IMPORTANTLY, 'WHY'?!

It is quite odd, I think, that people are shocked I didn't give up on life completely when I lost my sight. To me, it doesn't feel impressive. For as long as people have been saying that to me, I have been trying to explain the reasons why I didn't quit. It wasn't rocket science. It was simply down to the fact that it is a lot more interesting to live your life and enjoy the things that you do than to lie in your bedroom merely drifting through life. But, as a result of these questions, and perhaps for my own peace of mind, I have thought a lot more about the question of 'how' I have made the transition. This chapter contains my views on achieving the things that you aim for in life. It deals with the questions of 'what' our aims are and 'how' we achieve them. After we've talked about 'what' and 'how', I will look at the important question of 'why' we do things.

Over time, it has become clear to me that my own approach to achieving my aims is similar to the approach of many other people. In particular, I found that this applies to the people we have spoken to in preparation for writing this book. And while this chapter might be about achieving goals, the reality is that I did not just lie in my bed and set a list of goals for my life and a plan to achieve them. My progress has involved a constantly evolving process, much of the detail of which I certainly did not plan. But neither have I just lived my life from day to day without any regard for the future. I have set goals both for the specific projects that I have undertaken and for the bigger, more general, question of what direction I wanted to take in my life. Some of the things that I have done in the past just happened and I'm sure that some of the things that I do in the future will be unplanned too. On the other hand, some things I do plan. It is the same for the people we have interviewed and, I suspect, the same for you.

The 'What' and the 'How'

Making explicit your aims will certainly help you to achieve them. Sometimes setting a goal is more about telling people what you plan to do so that the information is out there – once you've said it then you are giving yourself the push to do it. It is not true that you have to write down your goals on a piece of paper and put them on your wall, although a lot of people do find that helpful. What is true, though, is that you will find your goals more difficult to achieve if you don't have some kind of vision of how to achieve them. You must at least have an idea of your overall plan so that you can make decisions based on some sort of knowledge of yourself. If one of your goals is to have fun for example, then you must know what activities you find fun and then do them.

For instance, a friend of mine called Jenny loved netball in school and she always talked about wanting to get back into it on a small scale. It wasn't something she set a goal for but she knew it was something that she would enjoy and that would keep her fit. When another friend came across a social league and mentioned it to her, she didn't hesitate. For someone that always prioritises enjoying her leisure time it was perfect. She knew that it was something she liked to do and it fitted into her overall desire to enjoy herself, to keep fit and to meet new people. She didn't have to set a specific goal, but at the same time she knew that it fitted into her overall plan.

Life can be very spontaneous and Jenny grabbed an opportunity on the spur of the moment to join something that she knew she would like. It's very important, I think, to allow these spontaneous things to occur in life, because, well, that's what makes life fun, isn't it? However, there is also a place, and I think a very big place, for taking charge of the direction of your life and for establishing a process that will allow you to gain satisfaction from your life. Certain things must be planned if we are serious about achieving them. In the following pages we will deal with those things that we attempt to plan in advance at different levels. Call it goal-setting, call it creating a mission, call it what you will. I have observed that successful people, once they are sure what they want, set out some kind of plan and that these plans have two broad levels.

The first I call the 'what', the second is the 'how'. 'What' are the overall objectives of our life? 'How' is the method we use to achieve these objectives. We have talked before about leading your life in a general direction by doing the things that you like, that you are good at and that are meaningful to you. After a while of following the right road, you will find that you want to speed things up, that you want to achieve certain things and that you begin to believe that you can achieve them. When this happens, you are starting to look at your life in a strategic way. When you are considering your life on a strategic level you are looking at the overall things that you want to achieve in your life, your great aspirations for yourself or your family or your business. In general, these are overall goals. When you are thinking about your overall aims you are thinking on a strategic level.

The 'how', which I also call the project level, focuses on tangible ends. If we acknowledge what we are attempting to achieve at a strategic level in terms of 'what', we can make sense of the 'how'. 'How' involves the nuts and bolts actions in our lives: the actions that we must undertake to bring us towards our strategic aims. Often, much of what we do at the project level of our lives is nothing to do with what really matters to us at the strategic level. There are lots of small projects that we feel we must undertake that have nothing to do with what we want. Too often, the things that we do are either dictated to us by someone or something else. I have noticed that when we are involved in projects that are mismatched to the things that we really enjoy, even if we have not explicitly identified those things, then we generally become disengaged and lack motivation.

The 'What'

Let's talk about the strategic level. This is the overall direction of our lives. These are the things in life that we hope to achieve in our lives. In our personal lives these could include many many things, like singing on Broadway, travelling the world, writing a book, earning lots of money, starting a family, becoming an entrepreneur or working in a multi-national corporation. In business, they include the direction that the company is taking or the direction of a particular team within a business. In sport, your 'what' might be to achieve an Olympic Gold or to be fit enough to catch up with your kids. The strategic level is all about our *modus operandi*, and thus should inform everything that we do.

At the time that I stopped studying economics in Trinity College Dublin and did my first talk in Shell Ireland I began a phase of introspection that still goes on today. The preparation for the talk was a little bit daunting. I had never done anything like this before and I had to speak for forty minutes. Forty minutes!

I had to think hard about what had got me out of bed in 1998 having gone blind and about how I ended up living a relatively normal life again. I had to communicate this to a group of people in a way that would have meaning to them so that they could apply it to their own lives. While it was interesting as an exercise in itself the process allowed me not only to review the series of rehabilitation projects that I had completed in the past – including working in my first job, completing a master's degree, starting to row again and so on – but also, more importantly, it prompted me to think about what really matters to me. It is this strategic level thinking that has resulted in what I am now doing in my life and the projects that I am now involved in.

Back in 1998, as I recounted in the last chapter, I had started a project with the aim of becoming an economist. But, at a strategic level, economics did not match enough of what I am about for me to persist with it. It was the start of another 'project' that I could have pursued but decided not to. Sure, I knew why I was doing economics. It was to develop some position in life that I aspired to, a profession that would pay me enough to live an extravagant lifestyle. But as I thought more about what mattered to me, prompted by the talk at Shell, meeting Miles, Caroline, Ian and reading the book by Charles Handy, I began to realise that my strategy was all wrong. Quite frankly, I hated what I was doing and I began looking to the future and asking myself the types of questions that have resulted in creating a framework for the projects I now undertake. For the first time I understood the importance of thinking strategically about my life. Now I know how important that is if I want to be happy in my life.

At this strategic level I began thinking about the things that make me tick. I looked at the things that I like and tried to bring them into a strategy. Strange as it may sound, earning large amounts of money did not feature as high on my agenda as it did before. Job satisfaction became much more important. I knew that sport and being fit were an important part of my life – for the camaraderie, the fitness and the competition – and I knew that I really enjoyed having time to go out with my mates, laugh with them and have a few drinks. Those were the things I enjoyed doing and as I thought about an ideal scenario for my life I knew I also wanted to travel. People ask me what I get out of travel, because being blind I can't really go sightseeing, can I? Well, it's really about being in new places, having new experiences and meeting new kinds of people. Sightseeing is well down on the list of priorities!

When I had thought it through, I came to the conclusion that the idea of doing economics with the aim of finding a job in which I would have to work long hours in a big bank doing something that I did not have a huge interest in simply did not make any sense. So why would I carry on with it? As I began to understand what really mattered to me, the next step was to try to work out a series of projects that included work, sport, travel, socialising and study that would facilitate me doing the things that I enjoy doing at a strategic level.

Now, the things I do – my career, my research, my sport and everything else – work in combination to define my life. What all of these things have in common is that they match my strategic goals. I have developed a business whereby I work with companies all over the world to develop the ability of their workforce to take decisions and make things happen, thus satisfying my desire to earn money, travel and interact with people. My sporting adventures combine travel with meeting people and help fuel my business as well as keeping me fit and providing me with great satisfaction.

My research in Trinity College Dublin mirrors the things that I do in my life and helps with all of my business and sporting strategic aims by complementing my experiential learning. The fact that I am doing research is a little surprising considering I did poorly in my school exams, failed first year in university and did a master's more to validate myself than for academic interest. Those facts seem strange, but now that I have found a subject that I am really passionate about (positive psychology and resilience theory) it is something that really excites me. My research is now more about learning and if I can use the learning to broaden my knowledge on the subject, then that will help my business because I will actually know my subject in much more detail.

You will notice that my strategic aims in 1998 did not include the pursuit of academic excellence for the simple reason that I never enjoyed studying. But now I do, and it happened as a result of pursuing the strategic goals that really did matter to me. The study started as a project to achieve my strategic goals by increasing my knowledge of my area but it is now sensitising me to the fact that at a higher level I do actually enjoy learning about human behaviour, psychology and the contexts in which we operate, whether that is in business, sport, politics, education or whatever else.

The reason I detail my experience is that at the time when I was attempting to understand what my strategic aims were, I had no real idea of how I would achieve them. But what I did know was that if I had a high level view of what mattered to me then I would at least have a chance of being involved in projects that I enjoyed and if I didn't enjoy every part of them at least I would know why I was doing them. Perhaps you question the things that you are doing sometimes. Do you have a satisfactory answer? Do you know what you are working towards? These are questions I might have had trouble with at one stage if anyone had cared to ask me. Knowing the answers to them certainly makes life clearer.

John, who we spoke about in Chapter 3, had a similar approach. He was working in San Francisco in advertising but he knew he wanted a change. He wanted to move back to Ireland to be closer to his family and he wanted to work in an area that he would find more personally fulfilling. On a strategic level he knew what he wanted, but he didn't rush into it. His first project was to travel around Europe and see what inspired him. He was on the look out for business ideas. He took the business ideas that he had seen in the United States and thought about applying them to the Irish market. Then, for another project, he volunteered at the Convergence festival for Cultivate, the sustainable living and learning festival. He was impressed by their enthusiasm and ideals but thought that he could add something different – he could apply some of what he learned in the US to their business and improve things. He thought that they needed more specific objectives and a more specific communication strategy. He thought that he could help them focus more and explain their story a little better. John has been there ever since, working in a job that he likes and believes in. He spent some time looking around for something that fitted in with his strategic goals and in the end he found it at the Cultivate centre.

In contrast, my friend Alex knew from early on that he

wanted to be a trader and work in a high stress, high risk environment. As early as when he was in school, he had being a trader as his target. Fast forward to the present day and Alex has been working as a commodity trader for the last eight years and is currently responsible for commodity derivative sales at Barclays Bank for Continental Europe and the former Soviet Union. He manages a team of eight people which is responsible for covering corporate clients who have, or would like to take, commodity (power, gas, oil, industrial metals, precious metals, coal, emissions [CO2] and freight) price risk in that region. He loves the fact that every day in his job is different and that he often has the opportunity to travel to places like China, Russia, India and Latin America. Alex is a great example of someone who knew what he wanted to do on a strategic level and pursued it until he achieved it.

The 'How'

All of the people that we have spoken to think and plan at a strategic level for their lives, their careers and businesses, but while thinking about what matters to you on a strategic level as a person or a business is important, equally important is making it happen. I have already explained my thinking on the difference between people who concentrate on making it happen as opposed to making excuses. John and Alex have thought strategically about their aims but they have also made the next step and pursued projects to move them closer to their strategic goals. I call this 'the project level of goals', the 'how' we achieve things, and this is when we move out of the conceptual part of goal-setting. It is when we take our head out of the clouds and concentrate on how we are going to make these concepts a reality.

For the project level I will first point out that the examples given are those of people who have thought about and understood what they are attempting to achieve at a strategic level. Therefore the examples given are of projects that complement their strategic goals and are moving them closer to their aims.

Alex, who I mentioned a moment ago, knew from an early age that he wanted to be a trader. I suppose many young lads give it a thought and imagine that it is an exciting career. Alex did, but he didn't just daydream about it and hope that it might happen, he set out to make sure that it happened. He worked out from the beginning the things that he needed to do to succeed. At school and in university he started deliberately building his CV by ensuring that he obtained the best work experience possible and by travelling. He even took a wine-tasting course at one point, much to the amusement of his mates. He knew what he was doing, though. Likewise, when it came to interviews he made sure that he knew as much about the companies that he was applying to as possible. These might sound like obvious steps but Alex told me that in university he was amazed at how few people actually pursued the thing they wanted in a deliberate manner. Alex knew 'what' he wanted and he figured out 'how' to get it.

Gavin, who we spoke about earlier, also developed a number of projects to help him achieve his strategic aim of getting into college to study medicine. It took him a long time before he decided that he definitely wanted to do medicine and there were a lot of good reasons for him not to do it, but once he had made the decision he started implementing a number of smaller plans to help him achieve his bigger aim. In the year and a half preceding his return to college to study medicine he developed the conditions necessary to ensure that he would be accepted into medical school and be ready to study when he got there.

Returning to college after you have become used to a substantial income cannot be easy. Gavin faced years of study at a time when most people have replaced serious learning with serious earning in their lives. Gavin would be watching his friends move further and further up the career ladder as he went deeper and deeper into his savings. He knew, though, that he wasn't happy in his job as a banker and when the opportunity arrived to change to a different job in a different company earning more money he jumped at the chance. In one way, he was investigating the possibility that he might change his mind about banking if he moved to another job. In another way he was implementing a project: earning and saving as much money as he could in preparation for returning to university.

The next project involved taking physics, chemistry and biology classes at the weekend so that he could pass the exam that medicine students must undertake to be accepted. He would work all day every day in his bank job and then spend the weekends in classes and studying. When he went for interviews in med school this was of great benefit to him. The doctors who interviewed Gavin seemed sceptical about him. They asked, 'why would a guy who is making a fortune and living the highlife in London want to return to college for years?' The projects that Gavin had completed showed that he was serious about what he was doing and he was accepted. Gavin's activities on a project level enabled him to get into university by giving him the knowledge necessary and also by convincing others that he was serious about what he was doing. His projects made him succeed on a strategic level.

In late 2002, around the same time that Gavin first applied to medical school, I was coming to grips with my strategic goals. That was when I first had dinner with Miles Hilton

Barber and it was from then on that things really gathered pace. During that dinner, Miles told me about his life. He was modest in the extreme and underplayed much of what he has achieved but lots of the things that he was doing in his life sounded so interesting and challenging to me that they changed my life and are greatly responsible for what I now do. In particular he told me of an event called the Marathon des Sables that he had taken part in. The event is a 250km footrace over the course of a week in the Sahara desert. It just sounded unreal that the blind guy sitting next to me, almost twice my age, had done such an extreme event but he kept telling me that I could do it if I wanted to and encouraged me to enter the race. Miles also told me of other adventures that he had done and how he used what he had learned on the trips to illustrate motivational speeches that he gave to companies. It was amazing because at the time I didn't really know any blind people, yet here I was sitting beside someone who I envied to the point of wanting to duplicate aspects of his life.

The stories of the Marathon des Sables stayed with me and, after a period of strategic thinking, it became a more and more attractive proposition so I visited the website for the race. The race was in April 2003 and, because it fell in the middle of the rowing season, it was impossible for me to compete in it. However, I did find an equivalent race to be held for the first time in the Gobi desert of China. Again it consisted of 250km, or the equivalent of six marathons in one week. Competitors had to carry all their own food, clothes, sleeping and survival gear. The race would be held in September 2003, after the end of the rowing season, so it not only worked with my plans for the year but it also meant I could probably persuade one of the rowers to guide me in the event.

In November 2002, ten months prior to the race, I decided

I would do it. I remember vividly what happened. I had pulled out of the economics course, I had done the talk in Shell and, really, the only thing I was doing was rowing. I wanted to run a business in the way that Miles did, speaking to companies and using adventures to teach things that they would find interesting and useful. As soon as I found the event I shouted over to my flat-mate, Nick, who was in the next room and let him know that I was doing the event. It didn't take long before Nick had committed to guiding me. Leading up to Christmas I informed everyone I knew that I was going to do the event and before I knew it one of my friends had contacted a couple of journalists about me and stories about our challenge started appearing in the weekend newspapers. I don't know if 'the goal' would have made it much further than the conception stage if I hadn't started telling people about it. After a while so many people knew about my project that I couldn't possibly change my mind. There was no way that I would change my plans and tell them all that I wasn't going to do the event. There was no turning back.

The Gobi March was a perfect project-level fit for what I was trying to achieve at a strategic level. I did not enjoy all aspects of it, either in the preparation or in the race itself, but I understood where the project slotted into the overall plan. In that regard it made sense even during the times that were difficult. The project goal was clear: the aim was to complete the 250km course inside the time allowed. How we did that is in the details and it is the details that are important for achieving project goals. We knew we had to complete six marathons in desert terrain in one week but neither Nick nor I had ever done even one marathon prior to starting the race, so we took all the advice we could get.

We calculated that if we had to be self sufficient for the

event then we would need the right food, so we tested different food and got advice from people who had raced in deserts before us. We were unsure of what medical care would be there despite assurance that it would be covered. So, we took responsibility for our own health and again took advice from others about what to bring. Specialist suppliers sponsored our clothing and again we took as much advice as possible. We even adapted some of our kit based on the advice that we had been given. Nick made 'gaters' out of parachute silk to keep the dust and sand out of our shoes in the hope that we might avoid the unavoidable – blisters. We took advice on training but the training was probably less of an issue because of the rowing training that we were used to. Although that was something we knew plenty about, there was much more we knew nothing about. The things that we knew about, we still took advice on, and the things that we didn't know about we took even more advice on.

The result was that we finished the race, we learned a lot about ourselves and I have been able to use the experience as an input to my business, my research and my life. The Gobi March was a goal at a project level that was so closely aligned with my strategic aims that the multiple benefits that have accrued from it are perhaps too numerous to explain in this book. I met people who I have since visited around the world, I have worked with others around the world, I have built and maintained relationships with sports companies and I am using what I have learned to take my research forward.

The Gobi March was a wonderful experience but also a tough experience. When it became very painful I had to remind myself that it fitted into my overall strategy and that kept me going. If you are clear in your overall strategy then you will find the right projects and stick to them. I have become much better, through time and experience, at keeping the overall strategy at the front of my mind and I am constantly looking out for new projects to help me achieve those strategic aims. The projects that I get involved in, some I enjoy, some are difficult and some I don't enjoy at all but they all are designed to move me closer to my strategic aims.

There is no rocket science in this. Once you are on the road of doing the things that you like and believe in, it simply follows that you should start to look more strategically at the direction you are taking. When you have a grasp of 'what' you want then it is natural to start considering the 'how'. There might be any number of projects that you can undertake to help you reach your strategic goals and finding them is up to you. There is no doubt an element of trial and error in this. In general you will have to seek out advice and help in making these projects happen. There will doubtless also be times when these projects seem difficult but remembering that they are part of the strategy will keep you going.

The 'Why'

If 'what' is the overall aims that we are striving to achieve in our life and 'how' is the projects that we undertake to achieve those aims, then 'why' is the question that we must constantly ask ourselves to ensure that there is a good reason for us having these aims. 'Why' is the question that enables us to maintain a course towards things that will give us satisfaction both in the short term and the long term. 'Why' is a question that gives meaning to the 'what' and the 'how'.

On the sixth anniversary of the day I lost my sight I had a telling lesson in 'why'. It was 10 April 2004 and I had just completed the North Pole Marathon. I was happy that I had managed to go from lying face down on a hospital bed to standing on top of the world in just six years, but I was disappointed with my level of competitiveness despite achieving my pre-race goal of completing the marathon. Another competitor, Sir Ranulph Fiennes, asked me the question: 'Well, what is it you are trying to prove?' It was a question that challenged me in a way that I hadn't been challenged since going blind.

In the last six years I've been ticking off boxes, achieving one thing after another in a step-by-step process to get back to where I was before I went blind. And along the way other people have been encouraging me, supporting me and praising me. The first challenge was getting out of bed. I did that. Great. I ticked off the box and got a pat on the back. Next was finding my way around the house, dressing myself and learning to read my watch. Later I moved on to living on my own, getting a job and doing a master's degree. When I was dealing with blindness as a possibility, I didn't know if I would be able to do any of these things.

I took a big step forward when I started rowing competitively again, winning medals for Northern Ireland at the 2002 Commonwealth Games, thus exceeding my previous achievements. At the same time I was developing my own business, which involved giving motivational talks to companies and individuals about overcoming obstacles and making changes. My new job was fusing my life's experiences with my business education, and completing extreme sporting challenges gave me great fuel for my talks.

Going to the North Pole was one such sporting challenge. Competitors don't touch dry land for the duration of the race, instead running on ice flows in -60°C temperatures just feet away from the vast depths of the Arctic Ocean. I fell at least ten times on my way to finishing the race, the deep snow leaving my face and hands frozen and sore despite my protective clothing. Unhappy at the finish, I asked myself: 'why am I annoyed despite having achieved the goal that I set myself?' Since then I have realised that I have not yet come to terms with certain elements of my blindness.

I had yet to accept that there are some things that I simply cannot do because I am blind. Prior to the North Pole experience I don't think I could have admitted that to myself and I would have viewed such an admission as defeatist. In the Gobi desert I ran six marathons in a week on rocky, ankle-breaking terrain but I didn't admit that my blindness held me back. Now I can freely admit that sometimes being blind does hold me back. I don't like it, but it's the truth. It has made me re-evaluate why I do things and I've realised how important that 'why' is. I will do more sporting challenges but before each event I will have to decide why I am doing that challenge.

I will aim to be competitive in events where there is a relatively level playing field for me. Other events I will do for different reasons and for other experiences. Understanding that I might not be competitive in a particular race, discipline or environment doesn't make me defeatist, it just means that the goal for that particular event is different. On each occasion the 'why' in the question, 'why am I doing this?' might be different. 'Why' links the 'What' and 'How' by providing a context for each goal. We must question our overall aims and the means by which we achieve them if we are to stay on course for achieving things that satisfy us.

Shortly after returning from the North Pole I read a book that further cemented my new thoughts on the question 'why'. The book was called *Man's Search for Meaning* and was written by Victor Frankl. A favourite quote of Frankl's came from Friedrich Nietzsche who said: 'He who has a why to live can bear with almost any how.' This quote summarises the message in Frankl's book and articulates the importance of knowing why you are doing things. If we can figure out 'why' we are doing things then we can ensure that our 'what' is correctly chosen and choose our 'how' in an intelligent manner.

Frankl went through the most incredible hardships in his life. His wife, father, mother and brother died in the concentration camps of Nazi Germany. Frankl himself came close to the same fate, enduring extreme hunger, cold and brutality, first in Auschwitz and then Dachau and facing the constant threat of going to the gas chambers. When Frankl entered Auschwitz all of his personal belongings were taken from him including a scientific manuscript that he considered his life's work. Despite all of this, Frankl managed to maintain his optimism and the conviction that his life still had meaning. He never gave up because he could always answer why he was living even if it was for the small things. His reasoning was that even in the most terrible circumstances, people have the freedom to choose how they see their circumstances and create meaning from those circumstances.

For Frankl the 'what' was survival, the 'how' was by maintaining his spirit and determination and the 'why' was the conviction that his life had, and would always have, meaning. If he didn't feel that his life had meaning then it would have been impossible for him to maintain his spirit and survive.

This is a very stark example and the categorisation of these questions are unlikely to be as straightforward in our own lives, but answering these questions is no less important for individuals whose lives might seem completely different by comparison. If your aim is to be an investment banker then it will help you to understand why that is your aim if you are to be able to maintain the desire to do that. It applies equally to an Olympic athlete or a student facing his/her final exams. Knowing 'why' you are doing something is the key to having a strong 'what' and 'how'.

*

If I think back to my life prior to going blind it is incredibly different to my life now and the answers to the 'what', 'how' and 'why' questions have changed completely. Back in 1998 I was about to graduate from college and had a job set up in London with an investment bank. In that final year in college I found myself applying for investment banking jobs mainly because they were considered the prestige jobs for business graduates. These jobs pay a large amount of money but for me, and I suspect for many of the other people, it is the prestige that goes along with getting the job that attracted me most. I applied for in excess of twenty-five jobs in London and half the time I didn't even know what I was applying for but in the end I was offered one job.

At that time I had a crystal clear idea of 'what' I wanted to do when I finished university and 'how' to achieve it. I knew that I wanted to earn lots of money and work in the finance world in London. I read a book called *Liars Poker* by Michael Lewis and another called *Rogue Trader* by Nick Leeson. Both books sold a high energy/high stress/big rewards lifestyle and I saw myself in that kind of environment. The 'how' of this aim was to apply for as many jobs as possible in an effort to increase my chances. It was a numbers game with me and I knew that if I applied for enough jobs that I would eventually get one. 'Why' was I applying for that job? The reasons were many: I was attracted to the money and the lifestyle and the respect I would receive from my peers. But I wasn't asking the question 'Why' strongly at the time and even if I had I'm not sure if I would have known how to answer it or even cared. In addition, I'm not sure if I would have been truly happy in that job, because the reasons I had for doing it were not particularly well thought out.

Now my life is very different to what it would have been if I had not lost my sight and had gone on to become an investment banker. Over time, and perhaps due to the shock of blindness and subsequent questioning of myself and everything around me, either my aims have changed or I have been able to understand what matters to me better than when I could see. Now I can answer the question 'why' and explain to you how that influences 'what' I do and 'how' I go about doing it. Can you answer these questions? Answering them will allow you to more easily achieve the things that interest you.

Main Points

- If you want to achieve your aims in life you must first make your aims known, both to yourself and others.
- If you want to achieve success, you must have at least an idea of an overall plan so that you can make decisions based on some sort of knowledge of yourself.
- It is absolutely key to take charge of the direction of your life and establish a process that will allow you to gain satisfaction from your life.
- Certain things must be planned if we are serious about achieving them.
- Think first about 'What' you want to achieve and then figure out 'How' you are going to achieve it.

- Once you have worked out your goals, you must go and make them happen. Nobody else will do it for you.
- To keep your life on the right course, consistently ask yourself 'Why' you are pursuing the goals that you are and ensure they fit in with what you want.

Try This Exercise

Exercise: Achieve your dreams

There is only one exercise to complete in this chapter but it is an important one.

First you must define and write down your overall goals in life. This is a list of 'What' you want to achieve. Write them down on a piece of paper. You might never have done this before but it is very important.

The next thing to do is prioritise them. Then take them one by one and we'll start to work on them.

Write your number one dream on another piece of paper and underneath this heading write down the steps that you feel you need to take to achieve them. These steps represent the 'How'.

Next, buy yourself a diary and start deciding when you can take each of these steps. What can you have done in a week? What will take you a month to do? Set yourself deadlines and figure out when you can complete each step. There might be ten steps to complete but if you take them one by one you will get there in the end.

Set yourself daily 'to do' lists and be methodical.

While big ideas are important and beautiful, success is in the details and if you work this way you will make it happen. Everybody I have met who works in this way finds success.

7
TEAMS – A NETWORK OF INDIVIDUALS

Most of what I have written so far is about me as an individual and you as an individual, but now I'm changing tack. I want to tell you about the experiences I have had that have convinced me that forming a team around you can be a big factor in achieving the things you are aiming for.

It almost seems to be a contradiction that a team can work for an individual because usually individuals work together to form a team. I've learned though that allowing others into my team can help me to achieve more things and achieve them much quicker. A good example of teamwork is this book. While the initial idea was mine and the connections and conclusions that I make are mine, I have recruited a friend to help me write it, and numerous other people to contribute their opinions, insights and experiences to the research. Without all of their help, I couldn't have done it.

Knowing what I know now, I am surprised at the reluctance of people, at all levels in society, to take an active part in putting people in place to help them achieve their goals. When I first started working for myself, I, too, thought I had to do everything on my own. In the beginning, I kept my ideas to myself for fear that others might steal them but soon

I started to meet more and more people who were successful and at the same time incredibly open. I began to reconsider my approach. I also noticed that they seemed to be able to call someone for advice on anything and everything. In short, it appeared that they were a member of a team.

There are all sorts of teams. People usually think of a sports team or a business team when the word is mentioned but the teams that these successful individuals were in were quite different to those traditional teams. They were flexible and constantly changing. In fact, there appeared to be different teams that they would plug into. And their teams were made up of all sorts of people. They might call their grandmother one moment for advice on cooking a dinner for a business client and then call an accountant the next to have the figures right for that same meeting. Their approach seemed much easier than mine. I had never considered teams in that way, but soon I began to and perhaps you could too.

A Formal Team

In my life there has been no team more formal than that of an eight-man rowing boat in a race. Even people who have absolutely no interest in sport will be able to understand the analogy. Perhaps you have seen such boats in the Olympics or at the Oxford University *v* Cambridge University Boat Race in England. In an eight-man rowing team there are eight rowers at the peak of their physical condition. These eight athletes are instructed by another person about half their weight, the cox, who sits at the back of the boat steering and making tactical judgements throughout the race.

A rowing eight is the archetypal team. It is eight individuals with individual tasks but their objective is to be as together as possible to achieve the aim of crossing the finish line first. Everybody wears the same racing kit, everyone moves as one and everyone listens to the instructions from the cox. For months the athletes train on the river and in the gym. For months they take advice from coaches, nutritionists and mentors. But as soon as the eight leave the pontoon in the final moments before their season's final race, they are on their own. Eight rowers and one cox – that is the team.

Back in 1997 I was racing for Ireland in the Home International Regatta in Nottingham. Four of my rowing team-mates from university and the cox were selected with four other guys from all over Ireland to make up an eight-man boat. In the eight, we were to race against England, Scotland and Wales. None of us was older than twenty-two at the time and most were much younger than that. Of the guys we were racing against many had 'been around' for much longer than us, or so we thought.

I remember pushing off the bank for our warm-up before the race. We were on a 2,000 metre rowing lake with only four boats on it. As we paddled away from the bank it was evident that we were completely together, as one. Everything that the cox told us to do was nailed in the warm-up and by the time we arrived at the start line all eight rowers were absolutely focused on our boat and what we could do to make victory happen. We left the bank for the warm-up like frightened rabbits in the headlights of a car but by the time we reached the start of the actual race I knew that everyone sensed the same thing as me. We knew we had a chance of winning the race and we just wanted to get on with it.

As we sat on the start line ready to go I felt almost sick with anticipation. From what I could tell, so did everyone else. When the buzzer went for the start of the race we exploded off the line. I was so pumped up that I wanted to blitz it from the start but the cox who was sitting in front of me was telling us to relax. 'Find the rhythm,' she said, 'on the rhythm, on the rhythm now.' She was forcing us to keep ourselves in control through the first half of the race, to hit the rhythm that we had felt in training and the warm-up. And that is exactly what we did. But as we came through the halfway point, with 1,000 metres to go, the plan was to take the race on. The cox called it: 'Now we're racing, this is our race,' she said. 'Ready … ready … go!' And everyone moved up a gear on her command. We were ahead at 1,000 and began to move away from the rest of the field through the 1,000 metre mark on the cox's command.

By halfway I felt fantastic or at least not dying a death like I have done in some races. As the cox called the push, my training and racing partner for the previous three years who was sitting directly behind me gave me the signal. He said, quietly but firmly: 'This is it Mark, it's ours if we want it, go!' We began to take on the race. In the position I was sitting, stroking the boat, it was my job to mark the rhythm for the stronger guys in the middle of the boat to apply their power. But from halfway on it was up to me to take it on and keep the boat moving as the rest of the guys began tiring. If I was fresh and was laying down a solid rhythm, they would have to go with me as I responded to the cox's calls. And that is what they did!

Again at 1,500 metres we took it up a gear but so too did England who had moved into second place. I knew they were finishing strongly but everyone in our boat was totally committed. We kept responding to our cox. She saw England coming at us and called for another effort: '500 to go, on the rhythm, on the rhythm!!' We took it up again. I could feel the other guys anticipate the line and the cox was driving us on, challenging us: 'Do you want this, do you want this?!!' She next shouted: '250 metres to go, ready … now.' We pushed again and again through the last 250 metres and crossed the line in front. We floated on, arms aloft and gasping for air, having won a race that we didn't think we could.

I don't think any of us really thought we could win that race before we went on the water for the warm-up. But we got on the water and stopped talking about it. Instead we concentrated on doing our jobs for the team. As the start line drew nearer, all our expectations rose. The energy in our boat as we sat at the start line was palpable. The commitment was unyielding.

Teamwork gave us victory over more experienced rowers and the strength of a team can be applied just as successfully to other elements of our lives.

A Different Type of Team

Rowing in that boat in 1997 was everything that a formal team represents – everyone with individual roles but all moving in the one direction. Let's just change our focus for a moment from sport to business. Think about the difference between a large multi-national corporation and a sole trader. Both approaches to business can be, and often are, extremely successful for the individuals involved. For the multi-national corporation with tens of thousands of employees much time and effort is put into the structure of the organisation, the business units, the teams and sub-teams. There is, in comparison to a sole trader, a large degree of organisation and it works well for many businesses.

Think of the big brand names that we see on any high

street, all of them have different layers of management and even more formal teams. Contrast that with a sole trader or an entrepreneur who is successful. Does an entrepreneur have a team or is he or she an individual? It is often difficult to understand who is working with, or for, a sole trader. The multinational is typified by structure and formal teams whereas the sole trader by definition employs nobody. However, a sole trader often must interact with a large network of people to be successful.

In the past I have worked in a 'traditional' job. I went to work Monday to Friday, performed a defined role and had a reporting line. Throughout my final months in university that type of organisation is all I wanted to be involved with. I craved a job in a prestigious organisation with a big salary and the opportunity to work my way up through the company. I wanted to get into a company that would allow me to operate in a defined team. Over time I have taken a different direction and now work for myself. As I think about what I do now, I have business relationships with many people yet I work for myself and by myself. Unlike the formal teams, such as the one that I described earlier in a rowing boat, we all have teams that are not locked into a boat or into a contract. We have people who we work with once, twice or even on a long-term basis, who disappear when we finish the project.

Let me go back to that race in 1997 at the Home Internationals again. I was trying to explain to you that rowing, once you leave the riverbank, is about who is in the boat. That was my formal team and the eight other people in that boat were my team-mates. However, it was the first and last time that I ever raced with some of them and apart from that one race it was the only time that this particular 'formal' team raced together. However, if I think about the others who helped me get to that point, the people who helped me to become selected for that boat and the people who helped me become good enough to contribute to the success of that formal team then other people come to mind.

My coach, Nick Dunlop, who I had been working with for the previous three years, was a part of the informal team that helped get our boat across the line in front of England. Nick was part of our team even though he wasn't at the event. Five of his athletes were in the boat and he had influenced us all. Four of us had been competing in a division of rowing that required us to be eleven stone or seventy kilograms. We had asked and received advice from people in universities, other experienced athletes and nutritionists. The other guys that we had been racing and training with that year, and longer, were part of the informal team. Without them we may never have been pushed on to compete.

Of course the eight rowers and one cox won that race in 1997. We were the ones who got the medals because we were the formal team. But I can count at least ten people who I would describe as being on my own team and I know that if I was to ask the other members of that crew to do the same, their answers would be similar. Yes, we are involved in formal teams but we must not lose sight of the importance of informal teams and networks that we operate in all the time. This applies not just to business but to our entire lives. The benefits of being in a team can be harnessed as much by a sole trader as it can by a sports or business team. I never would have thought that when I was a rower, funnily enough, but I am convinced of it now.

Informal Teams

In the course of writing this book, we have spoken to numerous people to get their views on the things that we have talked about. Whether they know it or not, they are part of the team of this book. There will be other members that will join when we go on to publish and distribute it. We couldn't have done this without their help. One of the people that we talked to about teams was a sole trader called Christina. She was mentioned in Chapter 4. Like most entrepreneurs, Christina works very hard. The day she came to meet us for a chat she had a pounding headache from the stress of work. For the last couple of years she has been running her own business, which involves designing and distributing accessories, particularly ladies' handbags. She started the business after her father died and left behind materials that he had used in the clothing trade.

Like anyone starting a business Christina has experienced ups and downs, but she certainly seems to be on the road to achieving her aims. And she is very happy in what she does. One of the difficulties of her job is that she works completely on her own, in her workshop. On the other hand, she has people around her who have been of help to her.

Christina's first major success came when she sold out at a craft fair. She had designed 250 bags and they disappeared so quickly that it was like magic. All sorts of people helped her in making that happen. She called on friends and family and other connections to ensure it was a success and it was. Without the help of others it might not have happened and she might not be in business at all. It was by telling people what she was doing that she started in the first place. Her first order came through a friend who she told about her business before she had even really started it. Since the beginnings she has had to build a network of people who can help her, whether it is by supplying her with necessary materials or by giving her a decent price for manufacturing her bags.

Christina made the point to us that people who are in business know how hard it is to get started. Most people who run a business have had to go through what you might be going through right now. In the same way, people higher up in your company have probably had to work at a lower level at some stage and know what it's like to have ambition. Some people like to keep those experiences to themselves, but many more are happy to provide help and advice to those who are on the same road as them but at a different point.

Building Your Team

Forming a network of people who you can trust and work with is about getting out and meeting people and finding out what they can do for you and what you can do for them. There are many ways of doing this. There are people and organisations out there that have realised the need for networking and have set up places where you can meet like-minded people and spread the word about your business. The Chamber of Commerce serves this function in many towns and is a good place to start. Often there are semi-state or local government offices that have an enterprise department which also aims to bring people together and to put entrepreneurs in touch with people who can help them.

It is not just entrepreneurs who need a team around them, although their need is particularly great. Everyone needs to have people around them who can give good advice. Even if you are moving to a new job or looking for a promotion within your company there are people out there who can help. The first port of call might be a family member or a good friend. But there also might just be someone in the evening course that you take who has been in a similar position and has a valuable piece of advice. Who knows, perhaps you are on your way home on the bus as you read this and the person sitting beside you has the answer to the question you've been asking yourself for weeks. Wait. Before you ask them, I should say that I'm not advocating speaking to everyone you meet. It's not natural for most people to do that, and it would certainly raise a few eyebrows. I am advocating not being afraid to discuss the aims that you have with people. Generally, people are very helpful, and you never know when you might be given a piece of advice that helps. One of the biggest aspects in forming a team is sharing with people what you are up to and being prepared of asking for help.

So often, in all aspects of our lives, we find ourselves in a position whereby we do not have all the answers. We attempt things that we find difficult to complete or things that we cannot complete without the help of others. That's not a bad thing. In fact, it's a great thing, because if you find yourself in such a position then it means that you are one of those people who is prepared to step outside of the comfort zone. Unless you are in that position on a regular basis in which case you are probably staying in your comfort zone.

I think that right from the earliest days of our lives we are forced to push the boundaries of our capabilities. Taking our first steps, going to school, riding a bike, living independently and getting a job – all of these things at one time were new to us, uncertain and different. But either out of necessity or choice we go and do them. Life requires us to try things by ourselves but more often than not we can benefit from the help, advice or encouragement of others. After all, none of us lives in a vacuum and when we do find ourselves in challenging situations, yes we must first look to our own resources and reserves but we do have the option to ask for help.

I remember, as a child, asking for help all of the time. If I couldn't do something or didn't understand something then the natural thing to do was to ask for help. It would be a rare child who could learn how to ride a bike for the first time on his or her own. Generally a relative will run alongside holding the bike in balance while the child pedals energetically. When the child feels that he has the hang of it, he shouts, 'Let go, let go!' Often it is only then that he realises that the relative has already let go. When we are youngsters, asking for help is natural. As we get older that seems to evaporate. There is nothing wrong with asking for help. We sometimes forget we can and, even when we remember, we sometimes hold back. Why is asking for help, or remembering that we can ask, so difficult?

One reason is that we fear imaginary consequences. Too often we worry so much about what might happen if we ask for help that we just will not allow ourselves to risk it. We sometimes fear undesirable consequences, especially from those with authority over us. Even when these fears aren't supported by actual data, they can be so strong that we risk giving up our goal rather than ask for help.

Asking for help removes any chance of us becoming the lone hero we so admire. If we ask for help we convince ourselves that we are diluting our own endeavour. We think that we must keep our success to ourselves yet being this way can actually stop us from achieving what we really want. Better to be a helped hero than a lonely failure. I remember for years having 'ideas' for different businesses. Almost all of them came to nothing because I was operating from a position of scarcity. I did not want to tell anyone my ideas in case they stole them. If I had shared my thoughts, perhaps my many ideas would be in the real world now rather than lost in my distant memory. If we become greedy and want to hog the glory to the exclusion of others we often stifle our progress forward. If you include people you trust you will have a team around you that can increase your chances of success.

Most of us were expected to work independently all through our education. To do otherwise was 'cheating'. We carry with us a sense that asking for help is a mark of inadequacy but, on the contrary, it is a strength to be embraced. Clever people within education often realise this. They're your classmates who form a study group. I remember seeing people doing this and thinking that it was a bit unnecessary and maybe even a little bit unfair. Looking back at it now, I realise that it is the smart thing to do. If you split the work you get more done and you can always, and yes I do mean always, benefit from other opinions and ideas. It is often said that the best film directors are the ones who are willing to listen to the ideas of the lowliest runner who makes the tea and directs traffic as well as consulting with the highest paid actor in the cast. Who knows where the next flash of inspiration might come from?

If we escape the barriers that hold us back from asking for help, we can put the power of asking into action with incredible results. By tapping into the expertise that surrounds us, simply by asking, we can put together a powerful team to help us make our aims happen. Let's talk about how we surround ourselves with the kind of people who can help us achieve our goals, the kind of people who can help us make it happen, simply by asking.

Everyone that we interviewed and many of the people who

we have spoken to while writing this book begin anything they do with an initial spark that comes from within. Nobody does anything with total commitment without some internal drive. In my own case, I was the only person who decided to get out of bed back in 1998, to start a computer course, to try to get a job, to go back to university, to start rowing again or to go to the Gobi desert or North Pole. Paddy was the only one who decided that he wanted to have a go at becoming a stand-up comedian. James was the only one who decided to get involved in coaching. Conor and Gavin were the only people that decided to pursue their medical degrees in different circumstances. Ger was the only one who decided to pursue his business interests as were Christina and Grainne and so on and so forth. I think you catch my drift.

All of these people were the ones who initially decided that they wanted to pursue the things they are now doing. But none of them has achieved any of their goals without the help of lots and lots of people. The way in which all of them have gathered their teams comes down to an ability to ask for help, to let others know what they are trying to achieve and to not be afraid of others knowing. All of the people in this book sooner or later decided that they were going to tell people what they were trying to achieve and were willing to ask for help, which has resulted in them getting there. Yes, they all feared the possibility that they might be rejected, that the person they were asking might say no. More often, though, people say yes, and help you to succeed.

As a politician, barrister and lecturer, Ivana probably couldn't do the wealth of things she does without the help of others. In politics you simply cannot be successful without the support of others. By definition, of course, you need votes if you want to hold office so you need the support of voters. In addition, you need the support of a wide network of professionals and volunteers to help you get the votes. Rarely have I met someone who seems so certain that they are doing the work they were supposed to as Ivana. She is deeply involved in working towards the goals she believes will improve society. In the work she does, she constantly calls on the help of a network.

A recent example was when she ran for the European parliament. She started with a group of people she trusts and works with regularly and began to build around that. From an initial campaign team of six people the team began to grow until there was a myriad of helpers on board. These kinds of teams are informal and many of the people are volunteers. They are also non-hierarchical to ensure that divisions don't occur. Everyone is involved and everyone is happy to be involved. They helped her to raise money for her campaign by organising numerous events. Ivana was amazed by how many people get involved and are prepared to help if you ask them

At the same time as that election there was also a referendum to amend the constitution in Ireland. In response to this Ivana plugged into another network. The group, 'Lawyers against the Amendment', started with a simple email to a number of lawyers and academics who shared a similar opinion. Before long a group of 200 like-minded people had grown from a small nucleus. Ivana is able to call on networks that have grown over time by speaking to people and by sharing points of view. She told us that it is difficult to ask for things sometimes but that when you are highly motivated by what you are doing then you are driven to do it. If you are motivated by something and believe in what you are doing, people will join in. You risk rejection, but there's more to lose if you don't ask.

Another one of our book team, Grainne, runs a business called Fruition that supplies high quality, artistically presented fruit baskets for all kinds of occasions. She's been at it for a few years and the business is growing gradually. She started it because she wanted to work for herself and had knowledge of the catering industry. She also wanted to apply her artistic flair. All of these factors came together in prompting her to launch Fruition. What she doesn't have is a lot of experience in running her own business. She has filled in the blanks by joining all sorts of business groups and not being afraid to ask for help.

One story is a particularly good example of what we are talking about. Grainne was a bit early for our meeting. She went to the lot to park her car and as she was at the gate searching for her pass when a young, beautifully-dressed girl from the car behind strode past her car and opened the gate for her. Grainne was taken aback. The girl seemed so organised and full of confidence. Because Grainne was early for our meeting, she decided to have a chat with this confident blonde-haired girl.

By coincidence, it turned out that Grainne had put a sales call earlier that morning to the bank where this girl worked. She worked in the marketing department and they discussed their different jobs. The girl told Grainne that her company spent thousands of euro a month on flowers and that she would consider fruit baskets in the future. Just by striking up a conversation and talking openly about her business, Grainne opened up the possibility of landing a big contract.

In my own case, if I think about my North Pole project the power of asking became more and more evident as the project persisted. Not long after returning from the Gobi desert, I was on a training run with a friend called John O'Regan. He told me about the North Pole marathon and by the time we finished the training run I had asked him to do the event with me. I didn't know how we would finance the trip, how we would cope with the conditions or even the reality of what those conditions would be. We started with one question and those few words began a series of events that culminated in racing a marathon at the North Pole on the sixth anniversary of the day I lost my sight.

It was John and I who did the race and the core team was just the two of us. But there were many more people in different areas involved in getting us to the race at the North Pole and these people were part of our team. These areas include training and nutrition, equipment, corporate sponsorship, charity fundraising and promotion. All of these areas involved many people, some that I knew well and others who I had never met. But anyone who got involved in the project did so because they were asked directly or became aware of our plans from other people who we had asked directly.

For example, all adventure runners face the problem of blisters and both John's experience of racing in the Sahara and mine in the Gobi desert led us to be hyper-sensitive about what shoes we should wear. However, running at the North Pole is not quite like running on a treadmill or even running in a desert or over mountains. Not only did we need to understand about which Gore-Tex lined shoes to buy, but we also had to take advice on the socks to get, as we needed to guard against frostbite. As it happened, our advice led to us getting two technical running socks that were extremely warm and also a neoprene shoe cover to stretch right over our waterproof shoes.

It didn't end there. As we could be running on ice and snow, some of which would be soft and deep, we began looking at and testing snowshoes. Like a modern day equivalent of the tennis rackets tied to the feet that you've probably seen in old movies, we brought two sets each with us to the North Pole and did our final testing in the days coming up to the race. We only decided what ones to buy having met and spoken with shoe specialists in adventure racing shops and having taken advice from previous snow-shoe racers. Buying shoes and socks might seem like a simple endeavour to you, but believe it or not we asked for help from eight different people. I'm glad we did, because our footwear worked out perfectly. After that we had to start asking people about food.

If you want to raise money you have to ask. Charities are always looking for money and one can learn a lot from trying to raise money for them. I have raised money for Sight Savers International on a few occasions. As you might expect, it is a charity that is close to my heart. I love the idea that I can in some way help others who are blind recover their sight. In the course of raising money for Sight Savers, I have asked so many people for help and I have received so much help as a result. Individuals gave money, companies gave money, voluntary organisations gave money and people I hadn't heard from for years got in contact.

A good example of what you can get when you ask came at a soccer match between Ireland and Australia in Dublin. When I heard that the fixture was on I called the relevant authorities and was given a permit to collect outside the ground and in the surrounding area. Sight Savers got buckets and t-shirts for people to wear while collecting and the next challenge was to get people to do the collections. I called lots of people, some who I had been in regular contact with and others who I hadn't seen for months and, in a couple of cases, for years. Thankfully most of them arrived ready to collect and some also brought friends. Nick got people out to collect, as did other people in my network of friends. Maybe thirty people were involved in that one collection and many of them had no reason to be there other than they had been asked and were willing to give up some of their time to help with our project. It was incredible and, from the charity's point of view, very profitable.

Asking people to collect was not the only thing that we did that day. The co-author of this book, Ross, rang the marketing manager of the Football Association of Ireland, Eddie Cox, to enlist his help. Ross asked Eddie if the announcer at the game could make an announcement to encourage people to donate. Eddie said no. He spoke at length about why he could not single out this particular collection because there were collections at every game. After he finished, there was dead silence on the phone. For a few seconds neither of them spoke. Then Eddie asked, 'So, what exactly is it all about?' When he had heard about why we were raising money and the lengths we were prepared to go to in order to raise that money he decided to help. I have never met Eddie, but I can only imagine that he is a very generous man. A big announcement was made at halftime in the game and it greatly helped our efforts. We asked him for help, and he in turn asked 50,000 people at the game for help.

*

I could write you a long list of individuals and groups that got involved in helping me in my sporting adventures, my business or my life. The one thing they all have in common is that they were asked to help in one way or another. Through this it became crystal clear to me how important it is to include people and to build a network of people that can help you and that you can help. I have been very impressed by the power of asking. For example in the Gobi March and the North Pole projects, all those who helped had been asked either by those directly involved in the project or indirectly by people who were enthused about what we were trying to achieve. Everything we did, from choosing shoes to wear to getting sponsorship to developing publicity and completing the event, would have been impossible if we hadn't asked for help.

I have worked on occasion with senior management teams and I am convinced that they need to ask for help in just the same way that I do when I get disorientated in the street and do not have my guide dog with me. When we need help, and we delay asking for it, we squander the most important resource that we have, which is time. What do you need help with right now? How soon can you ask for it? As soon as you do, you'll be starting to form your team. If you don't believe me, think about the things you have done that you feel really proud to have done. If you trace back how you achieved those results you will realise that you told people and asked for their help. As a result you drew on their experience and knowledge and that helped you achieve what you wanted. If you need help, just ask!

Main Points

- It almost seems to be a contradiction that a team can work for an individual but in fact forming a team around you can be a big factor in achieving the things you are aiming for.
- Teams are not limited to the arenas of sport or business – anyone who can provide you with help or support can be counted as a member of your team.
- When we are youngsters, asking for help is natural. As we get older that seems to evaporate. There is nothing wrong with asking for help.
- I've never met a person who could not benefit from some good advice from time to time.
- Forming a network of people who you can trust and work with is about getting out and meeting people and finding out what they can do for you and what you can do for them.

Try This Exercise

Exercise: Forming your team

Write down a goal in the middle of a page. Draw a triangle around it.

From one corner write the names of some people who are helping you achieve that goal in one way or another and the ways in which they have helped you.

In a different coloured pen and from another corner, write down some people who you have not asked for help, but who could offer you some kind of assistance in achieving your aim. Also write down what help they might be able to give you.

In a third colour, from the third corner, write down some related objectives that you need assistance with but have nobody earmarked for help.

Now, think hard about who might be able to provide that help. Draw arrows from names to activities.

On your page you have the basis of your team.

Some of the people you already know, some you might not have met yet. It's time to go and meet them and form your team.

Don't be afraid to ask for help!

8

PUTTING IT ALL TOGETHER

I STARTED WRITING THIS closing chapter on a trip to New Zealand to participate in an adventure race. On the trip I had an experience that reinforced in me the ideas that I have presented to you thus far. The truth is that I failed to complete the race and after the race I knew that I would have to go through all of the steps that we have talked about yet again if I was to make a success of it the next time around.

On the morning of 4 February 2005 I stood on Kumara Beach on the Tasman Sea with my team-mate, James O'Callaghan. Our intention was to compete in the Speight's Coast to Coast adventure race, a race recognised as one of the most gruelling multi-sport events in the world. We were about to traverse New Zealand's South Island by running, cycling and kayaking 243km of some of the roughest terrain New Zealand has to offer. Considering what I was about to face in the two-day event it surprises me now that I faced it with the composure that I did. It never crossed my mind at the time that we might not finish it and I wouldn't have entered the race if I thought I had no chance of finishing it. I had finished races in the Gobi desert and at the North Pole and I never imagined that this would be any different, but it was.

We started well, running the first 3km to the tandem bike

with relative ease and managing to stay out of trouble despite running in close quarters with hundreds of other athletes. Things were going so well that we even had time for a chat with some of the other athletes. The 55km road bike stage that followed was also enjoyable and we moved steadily through the field on our tandem. On the flat and downhill sections we carved through our slower competition and on the uphill portions we pushed hard and held our own. By the end of the cycle stage we were in the top half of the group and going well. We met our support crew, stuffed some food in and took on a mixture of energy drink and electrolyte fluid. Our cycling shoes were pulled off and our trekking shoes tied on. The transition was done in less than five minutes and then we hit the 33km mountain stage. Everything was going according to plan.

As we moved out of the transition point, away from the roadside and into the mountains, the screw tightened almost instantly. Before the race I thought that I would be running on the mountain stage although I knew there would be tricky sections with boulders where we would have to slow down and I would have to rely heavily on James for guidance. But the boulders were bigger than anything I had expected and the going was down to literally crawling speed at times. I had to totally trust James and another local runner who joined us called Josh Stevenson. We were stepping from boulder to boulder only as quickly as James and Josh could communicate to me where to place my feet and as quickly as I could respond. My responses became slower and slower as the day progressed.

By 2p.m., the temperatures had soared to the high thirties and I was becoming badly dehydrated. The terrain was brutal and I was beginning to trip more and more on the loose rocks beneath my feet. I was really losing concentration and eventually stopped sweating due to dehydration. Worse, I vomited after trying to take water on board. James and Josh must have been concerned at that point about whether I was going to make it. We had yet to make it to the top of the mountain and the time deadline was approaching fast. If we did not arrive at the top by the deadline, we would be disqualified. Mentally I was cracking and I knew it.

It was such a strange feeling. I knew that we had done a lot of the hard work and that if we got over the mountain it would quite literally be downhill all the way to the finish line for Day 1 of the race. But we had only completed 16km of the 33km mountain stage. It was clear that we had not moved quickly enough and that we would not be allowed to continue due to the time cut-off. I was crushed when I considered the prospect of being helicoptered from the mountain but, at that point, deep down I knew I wanted the pain to end. My mind was saying 'don't admit defeat ... you are being soft ... you are taking the easy way out'. We had no choice but to stop. We admitted defeat and flew from the mountain to the finish line by helicopter.

It was both devastating and humiliating to arrive at the bottom of the mountain and leave that helicopter to the applause and cheers of fellow competitors at the finish line. We even got an award for 'best effort' at the award ceremony. I understand that people were empathising with us for our efforts but neither James nor I went to New Zealand to not finish the race. It is the first event I have not finished and I hate the fact that it happened. It is a failure and I cannot see it as anything but a failure. I did not enter the event with the intention of not completing it, yet that is exactly what happened.

Reacting to Failure

As far as I can work out, there is no such thing as a life without failure. We have all failed at one time or another. It's not fun, and I think my story is a testament to that. Try as we might to avoid failure, it will happen to us at some point. The way in which we react to failure is the important thing. Considering this point and planning for next year's race has taken me through the steps we have talked about in this book all over again.

When I read through the stories in this book and think of the conversations I had with people while writing it, I realise that all of these people have failed at one time or another. But I have also realised that the people in this book do not dwell on failure. Instead, they draw a line in the sand, accepting their lot and looking to the future. Acceptance was one of the first things that we mentioned in this book and accepting failure and moving on is key in guaranteeing future success.

I failed to complete the Coast to Coast race and that was not a fun experience, I can tell you. However, quickly thereafter I accepted the fact. Perhaps I could have blamed someone else for the failure or skulked around feeling sorry for myself, and perhaps I was even a little bit tempted to, but soon I realised that if I wanted to move on and have success in the future I would have to accept the defeat, analyse it and start taking steps to make sure I was successful the next time. The same tools that I used post-sight-loss could be used in this scenario and I began to do that.

Trying to shy away from the reality of what has happened will not change the experience. Blindness, the Coast to Coast race and all of the other challenges in my life I now deal with in this way. It is the only way. Blaming other people and being angry about the result are not going to change it. And feeling sorry for myself is not going to turn the clock back and reward me with a second chance. Only by accepting that it has happened can I even consider moving on.

To move on, I will start by taking the first steps. Those steps will be making a plan that will give me a much better chance of completing the race next year. Once the plan is in place I will set goals and begin to make it happen by achieving those goals. I will form a team around me to give me advice on preparation, to help me raise money for the event and to support me during it. I know that I will persist with it because I know that the reward will be great in the end and in a year's time I'll be ready to give the Coast to Coast race 2006 my best shot.

Go for it!

There is another story that I want to tell you that I hope will encourage you to really go for it and start making changes now that will improve your life. That decision is one of the most important that you will make in your life. This story is about my recent efforts to learn how to dance. I have done some pretty frightening things in my life but I have never feared anything as much as dancing! I remember even from an early age I feared dancing beyond all reasonable proportions. Any mention of dancing at a social gathering was my cue to get the hell out of there.

Yes, for most of my life I consistently avoided dancing at all costs. I cringe now at some of the situations that I found myself in. For instance, in university I was at a ball with a girl whose friends I did not know very well. I sat through a four-course dinner and listened to all of them chipping in about how much they were looking forward to the dancing that would follow. None of the others seemed to have my deeprooted fear and as a result they seemed to have no interest in building up their confidence through wine consumption. I was crying out for a drinking partner in crime but there was none. These people were dancers, not drinkers. I had to hold back because even I knew that I wouldn't impress this girl if I drank all of the bottles of wine by myself.

Dessert came and was scoffed. As the coffee was poured I was becoming increasingly irritated and worried. Soon, people began to mingle and chat. The atmosphere was building and I could feel people were revving up for the dance-floor. Then, out of the corner of my eye, I noticed a friend who had an equal, and joyously similar, fear of dancing. Within seconds we had bolted and spent the rest of the night in the bar adjoining the ballroom happily chatting and drinking, safe in the knowledge that we were in the furthest position possible from the dance floor. Phew, another dance disaster had been averted.

In June 2004 I was on a speaking tour in Australasia and travelled back to Ireland via New Zealand where I met up with a friend who had been travelling in the region. We flew together to Fiji and then on to a smaller island. As soon as we stepped off the plane, the sounds of South Pacific islanders' music filled the air and the first dance of the trip was forced upon us when a lady in the airport put shell necklaces around our necks. Nick and I were put in the middle of a circle and designated as spokesmen for our tourist group. Happy with our new found status and on an island of thirty people we were delighted to drink the Cava, respond to prompts from our hosts and sit while the islanders performed local war dances in front of us. The guys seemed to just stamp their feet and the girls (according to Nick) danced in a manner that meant that their stomachs stayed completely still while everything else moved as if completely detached from their bodies.

We stayed on the island for five nights and had great laughs with the other people staying on the island. We kayaked and swam during the day and ate with the locals and the visitors at night. While the dinner and drinks were fun, we were soon left abandoned at the bar and as we stood there everyone else danced. In Ireland, it is the bar that is busy, in Fiji, it was not. Dancing, it became evident, was our only way to get involved. And we did. War dances, fire dances, dancing around the bonfire on the beach. By the end, you quite simply could not stop us. I remember one night heading off dancing and by the time I came back Nick was decked out in a sarong and shell necklace. I, on the other hand, had promptly bought a shark's tooth to hang round my neck. We had become fully paid up members of South Pacific island dancing society!

We then travelled through California, dancing with girls in night-clubs and, on one memorable night, on the street in San Diego. We plucked two girls from the queue outside the night-club and danced with them in the street. I don't know what happen to Nick but I had to give mine back when her boyfriend asked me to. Finally we travelled to Miami Beach where I was delivering a talk to the Miami Beach Chamber of Commerce. The talk went well and Bruce Singer, the then CEO of the Miami Beach Chamber, asked us what we wanted to do while in Miami Beach. Everyone we had met had told us to go to a night-club called Mangos in Miami Beach. In a few minutes the guy had made some calls and had a table reserved for us at the venue. Buoyed by our dancing success in Fiji and San Diego, we were primed and ready for Mangos.

Arriving early, we got our seats and Nick started describing the dancing that he could see taking place on the dance floor. Initially there was only one couple dancing but another soon joined them. He said that it looked like a demonstration by professionals. According to Nick, the girls seemed to have similar skills to the Fijians in keeping their stomachs completely still and shaking everything else. The Latin American and Cuban music was pulsing and the atmosphere was electric. I'm not sure, but I think at one point Nick fell off his chair with the events that were unfolding.

Before long, everyone was dancing and the place was packed with people who were all doing a dance that we simply could not match, despite our previous two weeks of building the skills! We stayed there from seven in the evening until five the next morning and tried to pluck up the courage to dance. The place was packed yet the only girls we managed to talk to were the ones behind the bar when we ordered our drinks. It was clear that dancing was the only route to speaking to anyone in Mangos.

On the plane home, I decided that I wanted to learn to dance. I searched the internet and found some dance classes for Swing, French Jive and Salsa. All I wanted to do was to learn to dance enough so that I would not embarrass myself in situations where dancing was compulsory. Not long after returning from Miami I bumped into a friend of a friend in Dublin who dances. I told her about the Miami experience and asked where it would be best to learn. She gave me a couple of names of places and even said she would show me some basics if I wanted. Over the next couple of months I went to a class in Dublin with Nick and a couple of others. French Jive was the name of the style and our only criteria was to be able to spin girls around in a night-club or at a wedding. French Jive seemed to hit the spot. For one night we were spinning and spinning and dancing girls off the dance floor. It was brilliant and because everyone was a beginner the fear factor was reduced. Everyone was terrible. But that is why we were there.

That class ended abruptly the next week when the teacher called to say that he was living too far away from Dublin and that he was not going to commute anymore. It was a false start to my dancing career but I wasn't going to give up. I emailed the girl who had originally given me the dance contacts. Her name is Simone and she dances salsa and she agreed to teach me. She came over to my kitchen and played some of the music. It was exactly what we had heard in Mangos in Miami Beach and as she began to teach me it was clear the dancing that Nick had described to me was the dancing that Simone was teaching me. Brilliant!

Since that first class I have danced with Simone in my kitchen and in loads of clubs in Dublin. The funny thing is that I persisted for twenty-eight years knowing that I would have that fear every time I was faced with the prospect of dancing. In the space of two weeks as I travelled through Fiji, California and Miami Beach I decided that I didn't want to do that anymore. Now I have discovered that I actually really enjoy dancing, have made new friends and revived old friendships. In many ways I wish I had done it sooner. My experiences while travelling really prompted me to go for it and I'm so glad that I did.

Dancing on the face of it is not exactly the cutting edge of seemingly 'serious' decisions that we all make. But the kind of decisions that I make in my business, my sporting pursuits and my life are fundamentally comparable to those that I made in the story I have just told you about dancing. It's amazing what you can achieve in all parts of your life when you really go for it.

The Importance of Attitude

Just after I wrote that last section I paused for a break. I was sitting alone in a hotel room in Hong Kong and began to reflect on my day. It began when I travelled by myself from my hotel room in a foreign and strange city to a meeting with the CEO and human resources director of a company that has 220,000 employees in the wider group. Later, I had another meeting over lunch and in the evening I spoke to a small group of fifteen people who are, between them, managing US $18 billion. It had been a long day in Hong Kong and I had done all of these things on my own. I sat there, tired, thinking that it had been a very good day and that I had achieved a lot.

As I sat there in my hotel bedroom I was immediately transported back to another time, and another bedroom. Suddenly, I was back in 1998 when I first went blind and I could not help but make comparisons. The previous few days were so far removed from the time in 1998 when I had sat in my bedroom unable to go downstairs or set an alarm clock. I had felt bombarded with a certain sense that it was okay for me to make excuses as to why I could not live the life that I wanted to now that I was blind. I was also faced with a myriad of services charged with rehabilitating me back into society. Some were necessary and fantastically helpful but when it came to my job search I faced a serious barrier and it was one of attitude. As helpful as some of the organisations were, they seemed to spend a lot of our contact time telling me all of the things that I wouldn't be able to do.

I was being encouraged, it seemed, to have an attitude that wouldn't help me to achieve the life I wanted. One result was that I felt I was going to be a useless human being due to my blindness. Another was that I did not think I would be able to contribute in the workplace or in society. Some of the people I came into contact with, especially when it came to my job search, were more than happy to force the excuses upon me. It felt to me as if they almost wanted to highlight the blindness so that in some way I might have an excuse not to even try.

Yet now I am working and travelling and making decisions for myself. The excuses I could have used either by choice, or because I didn't know any better back in 1998, are no longer there when it comes to my blindness. Instead they are replaced with solutions. Sometimes those solutions manifest themselves in the form of other people's help and sometimes they are aids that I use, like my computer or my dog or my white stick or braille watch. The biggest solution, however, is in having the right attitude. The right attitude will allow you to stop making excuses and instead, make it happen.

It took me a long time to deal with my sight loss but I now rarely even think about it. When I think about what I have just done in these few days here in Hong Kong it is clear to me that my attitude has changed over the last number of years. Without a shadow of a doubt I could have decided not to come to Hong Kong on this trip. I mean, how could a blind person fly from Ireland to Hong Kong without a travelling companion? The answer: ask for help and get the taxi driver to pass you to the airline staff who will then pass you to the bus driver who passes you to the hotel staff. Yes you need to trust people and you have to take a risk but if you do it you are suddenly in Hong Kong, less than twenty hours after leaving your door in Dublin.

How would I give a presentation at a dinner in front of a small group of heavy hitters in the financial world? I prepare to do it and practise the talk. How would I set up a business meeting? I get a computer that talks back to me and email the companies, arrange the date and time, confirm on the phone and get the hotel staff to leave me to a taxi and get the building attendant to meet me at the other end. And finally finish writing a book? Well that comes down to my mind and my computer and deciding to write it with a person who can write and edit the work!

Attitude is a choice and as I have worked with more and more people in the corporate, sports, education and personal development arenas I have been confronted with the contrast between people who have an attitude that allows them to make it happen and those whose attitude prompts them to make excuses. Often the people with the attitude to make it happen have been practising it in one or many parts of their lives. They have chased their goals and gone after what they want with gusto. I have also met people who pursue, with the same energy, the practice of making excuses. Having the right attitude can transport you from one camp to the other.

Take Control and Achieve Now

You can change your attitude quicker than you can change your clothes. You can change your attitude right now, in a second. The challenge then is to keep it the way you want it. In this book I have outlined the step-by-step process that I took to go from someone who was faced by many excuses to someone who now makes things happen in my life. If I can do it, you can do it too. That I promise. Once you change your attitude and decide that you are going to make things happen in your life then you are taking responsibility for making your dreams happen, whatever those dreams might be. If you change your attitude then you are taking control. Who better to be in control of your life than you?

To learn more about Mark Pollock's
speaking business and associated products, go to:

http://www.markpollock.com